CONTRACEPTIVE DILEMMAS

CONTRACEPTIVE DILEMMAS

Second Edition

Anne Szarewski MBBS DRCOG PhD MFFP FFFP
Clinical Consultant, Honorary Senior Lecturer
Cancer Research UK Centre for Epidemiology,
Mathematics and Statistics
Wolfson Institute of Preventive Medicine
London

ALTMAN

Published by Altman Publishing, 7 Ash Copse, Bricket Wood, St Albans, Herts, AL2 3YA, UK

First edition 2003
Second edition 2006

Typeset in 10/12 Optima by Scribe Design Ltd, Ashford, Kent
Printed in Great Britain by Ingersoll Ltd, Wembley

ISBN: 1 86036 035 1. ISBN-13: 978 1 86036 035 0

A catalogue record for this book is available from the British Library

∞ Printed on acid-free text paper, manufactured in accordance with ANSI/NISO Z39.48-1992 (Permanence of Paper)

CONTENTS

PREFACE

This book adopts a problem-based approach. I have used my experience of questions commonly asked during lectures, practical training and in general discussion with colleagues from both the medical and nursing professions. Where possible, I have included evidence to support the management options suggested. I hope this approach will appeal to family planning doctors and nurses, general practitioners, gynaecologists and healthcare professionals in related specialties.

My aim is that *Contraceptive Dilemmas* should provide a useful and quick reference for those involved in providing reproductive healthcare in many settings. I have not set out to create a resource for clinicians hoping to start from scratch in their reading on contraception, but aim to provide practical information for those who are faced with contraceptive problems in a clinical setting. In addition, I have included a section on new products, in order to keep practitioners abreast of developments.

The evidence base for the provision of contraceptive care is constantly changing. I hope that this book provides the reader with some useful information and ideas. For interested readers I would recommend the Faculty of Family Planning and Reproductive Health Care website (www.ffprhc.org.uk) where they will find recommendations for clinical practice and researched summaries of evidence pertaining to questions sent to the Clinical Effectiveness Unit (CEU). There are also other sources of reference, such as Bandolier and the Department of Health website (www.doh.gov.uk). This has statistics on every subject, including cancer, abortions and births and government health news (e.g. the Teenage Pregnancy Strategy document). It also provides links to an array of government-related organizations, including the Medicines and Healthcare products Regulatory Agency (MHRA).

In this new edition, I have updated most of the sections as new evidence has emerged. I have also included more references so that interested readers can check original sources more easily. Thus, I hope the book is as up-to-date and evidence-based as possible. It remains sadly true that in many areas I do not have definitive evidence and have to rely on a critical assessment of what is available. It is to be hoped that more, good quality research will be carried out in this field.

AS

PART 1

CURRENT ISSUES IN CONTRACEPTION

1 COMMON MANAGEMENT PROBLEMS WITH COMBINED ORAL CONTRACEPTIVES (COCS)

Problems such as weight gain, breast tenderness, headache, mood changes, breakthrough bleeding (BTB) and acne are often referred to as 'nuisance', 'subjective' or 'minor' side effects, but have an important influence on COC acceptance and continuation rates. Women are more likely to stop taking the COC pill because of such 'minor' side effects than because of worries about potential health risks (International Working Group on Enhancing Patient Compliance and Oral Contraceptive Efficacy 1993). When prescribing the COC, healthcare professionals tend to focus on what we regard as health risks; however, if effective contraception is the aim, then we must ensure that patients' concerns are also dealt with to their satisfaction.

Weight and bloating

Concerns about weight gain act as a disincentive to COC use for some women. The published literature does not provide convincing evidence that the COC causes weight gain, but is hampered by difficulties in study design (Webb 1996). It is likely that, for the majority of women, the COC does not cause weight gain, but is blamed for the natural tendency of people to put on weight over a period of time. Nevertheless, some women certainly feel bloated when taking the COC and it is possible that it contributes to weight gain in certain cases.

Acne

Acne and hirsutism are difficult to study scientifically, but clinical experience has for some time supported the beneficial effects of third-generation progestogens in these conditions (Levrier *et al.* 1989; Erkkola *et al.* 1990; Mango *et al.*1996; Redmond *et al.* 1997; Walling 1998). It has long been a problem with second-generation COC pills that if a woman suffers from both BTB and acne, it is very difficult to improve both conditions at the same time. BTB is improved by the use of more progestogen, or a more potent progestogen. However, if the progestogen has androgenic effects, this will almost certainly make the acne worse. The use of the less androgenic, third-generation progestogens has been an enormous help in such cases. Dianette (ethinylestradiol 35 μg and 2 mg cyproterone acetate) is licensed as a treatment for acne and hirsutism, rather than a contraceptive. However, it is a perfectly effective contraceptive as well. It is recommended for use in the presence of moderate to severe acne and can be used as long as the acne continues to improve, changing to another brand if there is no improvement or the acne resolves.

The new COC, Yasmin, has been shown to be as effective as Dianette for women with mild to moderate acne (Van Vloten *et al.* 2002). Thus, for women whose acne falls into those categories, it might be reasonable to use Yasmin instead. Otherwise, Dianette could be continued until the acne improves, and the patient then switched either to Marvelon, Yasmin, Cilest or one of the other skin-friendly COCs.

Management of breakthrough bleeding

Breakthrough bleeding (BTB) is defined as bleeding other than during the pill-free week. BTB is not uncommon, especially in the first few cycles of COC use (up to 30%) and can vary between being heavy and spotting. The latter can cause a dark brown discharge, which causes concern to many women. In the majority of cases there is no significant underlying cause. It is, however, important both to warn women that it can occur and also to ensure that appropriate investigation is carried out when indicated.

A woman presenting with breakthrough bleeding should have a history taken and if necessary be examined and have further investigations. BTB that occurs after a period of time without problems or that is persistent is more likely to be significant. Box 1.1 indicates the commoner causes of BTB. Correct pill taking should be checked; if pregnancy is possible a pregnancy test should be carried out. Do not forget that another healthcare provider, such as A&E or Genitourinary Medicine, may prescribe your patient other medicines. Some drugs may reduce the efficacy of the COC or lead to BTB (see 'Drug interactions').

Box 1.1 Causes of breakthrough bleeding

- Forgotten pills
- Vomiting or very severe diarrhoea
- Drugs
  broad-spectrum antibiotics (penicillins or tetracyclines)
  enzyme-inducing drugs including some antiretroviral drugs
- Pregnancy
- Infection
  chlamydia
  pelvic inflammatory disease (PID)
- Malignancy
  cervical cancer
- Malabsorption
- Distress
  the 'weeping womb' syndrome
- Diet
  vegetarians often seem to need a higher dose pill
- Dose

Given that the majority of pill users are young women, the possibility of a sexually transmitted infection such as chlamydia should be borne in mind. This does not mean that every woman with BTB should be extensively investigated, but it is worth bearing those factors in mind, especially if she has persistent BTB.

Specific conditions require appropriate management. Recent-onset BTB with no significant underlying cause can be monitored and the patient can be reassured that this does not indicate reduced efficacy of the COC. There is no dogmatic way to manage other cases of BTB, although it is usual to empirically try other COC preparations. This is not totally without science but a positive outcome cannot be guaranteed.

Third-generation COC pills have been reported to give better cycle control, with fewer reports of BTB in the early months compared with second-generation COC pills (Loudon *et al.* 1990; Brill *et al.* 1991; *Drug and Therapeutics Bulletin* 1992). A British multicentre double-blind study (Loudon *et al.* 1990) compared 189 women taking Femodene

(30 µg ethinylestradiol with 75 µg gestodene) with 185 women taking Microgynon (30 µg ethinylestradiol with 150 µg levonorgestrel) for 6 months. There was less BTB present in the first three cycles (17% for Femodene compared to 28% for Microgynon) – a time when many women discontinue their contraceptive method, particularly if they have so-called 'nuisance' side effects (Belsey 1988; Hillard 1989).

Studies have shown that if 10 different women are given the same pill at the same time of day, 3 hours later blood hormone levels will vary widely. This suggests that some are absorbing less or metabolizing faster than others. If that is the case, then the women with BTB need more hormone to reach the same blood level than the women who do not have BTB. They are unlikely to be put at greater risk of side effects or health risks, because their hormonal blood levels are the same. If a woman does have BTB, and it looks as though it is just down to the dose, it is best to increase the dose of the progestogen initially; if that does not work, an increase of oestrogen dose may be tried. It is unfortunate that we no longer have higher dose pills, containing 50 µg of ethinylestradiol. Although it is likely that the presence of BTB indicates a different rate of metabolism in that individual and that increasing the dose is safe, there are no specific safety data on this and the slightly controversial method of prescribing two packets of low-dose COCs to be taken simultaneously to make a higher dose is outside the product licence.

Breakthrough bleeding occurring regularly in the first week of the packet can sometimes be remedied by shortening the pill-free week, perhaps to 4 days instead of 7. Sometimes a triphasic pill helps to settle the bleeding pattern without having to resort to a higher dose, but this may lead to premenstrual-like symptoms as the hormone levels change.

Here are some suggestions for dealing with BTB on specific pill formulations:

- Best cycle control is given by Minulet/Femodene. Cilest, Marvelon and Yasmin are all roughly similar and not quite as good as Minulet/Femodene. Femodette and Mercilon are at the bottom of the list, although the difference between them and Cilest, Marvelon and Yasmin is not great.
- BTB on Mercilon, Marvelon or Cilest (there is not enough difference between them to warrant changing from Mercilon to Marvelon): change to Minulet/Femodene. If this still does not work, a triphasic sometimes helps.

- BTB on Ovysmen/Brevinor (which contain 35 μg of oestrogen, plus 500 μg of norethisterone): BTB on this formulation is common. Equally common is to miss withdrawal bleeds, especially if the woman has had BTB. A change to Marvelon or Cilest is usually enough, and if that is not successful, follow the rules for BTB on Marvelon.
- BTB on Microgynon/Ovranette (which contains 30 μg of oestrogen plus 150 μg of levonorgestrel): this is unusual, but if it occurs, try Minulet/Femodene first. If that is unsuccessful, a new triphasic may help.
- BTB on older triphasic pills (Trinordiol/Logynon/Logynon ED, TriNovum/TriNovum ED): one of the newer triphasics, such as Tri-Minulet or Triadene may be enough. Or try Minulet/Femodene.
- BTB on Neocon (35 μg of oestrogen plus 1 mg norethisterone acetate) or Loestrin 30 (30 μg of oestrogen plus 1.5 mg of norethisterone acetate): if this occurs, Minulet/Femodene is a possibility, but cannot be guaranteed to be strong enough.
- BTB on Loestrin 20 (20 μg of oestrogen plus 1 mg of norethisterone acetate): this is almost universal, which is why this pill has never been very popular. A change to Mercilon or Femodette will probably be enough.

If all the new pills are not available, as a general guideline, BTB on Marvelon, Mercilon, Femodette or Ovysmen/Brevinor will often resolve with Microgynon/Ovranette. If not, try either Loestrin 30, or Neocon.

Migraine

Migraine is an independent risk factor for stroke, with the effect being greatest in women suffering from migraine with aura. The aura comprises focal neurological symptoms, which usually precede and resolve before onset of migraine headache and associated symptoms. Visual aura is the most common symptom, occurring in 99% of auras, and will most commonly be tunnel vision, loss of half a field of vision, or fortification spectra. Note that generalized 'flashing lights', blurring of vision and photophobia are not considered to be suggestive of focal ischaemia (MacGregor 2001). Sensory and motor symptoms can occur but are less common. They have a unilateral distribution, often in the face or arm. The effect on stroke is increased further in COC users; in general, the following groups can use progestogen-only methods, but should not use the COC:

- women who have migraine with aura;
- women who develop severe or recurrent migraine for the first time whilst using the COC;
- women with frequent or severe migraine;
- women with simple migraine together with other additional risk factors for arterial disease, e.g. heavy smokers with a strong family history of arterial disease.

Simple headaches

Simple headaches and migraines may both be aggravated by water retention and therefore less oestrogen, or progestogen dominance is usually the answer. If they occur only, or to a much greater extent, in the pill-free week, the woman should be advised to tricycle.

Headaches or migraines occurring in the last week of a triphasic pill will usually be improved by the use of a monophasic pill. If there is still a problem and all the above suggestions have been tried, the general rule is to try the lowest-dose pill possible that does not result in BTB.

Drug interactions

Drug interactions potentially affecting contraceptive efficacy

All but the most obviously symptomatic drug interactions are difficult to identify, and there is widespread under-reporting of suspected adverse drug reactions. Wide inter- and intra-individual variations in circulating hormone levels complicate the picture. Pre-marketing clinical research on new and established drugs will often exclude women taking COCs, and well documented experience with many thousands of women-years of use is necessary to demonstrate uncommon interactions. The clinical significance of identified *in vitro* changes is often difficult to establish.

Drug interactions may occur at any stage between absorption and excretion. The most clinically relevant contraceptive-impairing interactions are with anticonvulsants and broad-spectrum antibiotics, which

I summarize here, more detailed guidance is available from the Faculty of Family Planning (Faculy of FP 2005).

Liver enzyme inducers

Hepatic enzyme-inducing drugs such as anticonvulsants (e.g. phenytoin, barbiturates, carbamazepine), anti-tuberculous (rifampicin), antifungal (griseofulvin) and some drugs used in highly active antiretroviral treatment (HAART) will increase the metabolism of the COC and the progestogen-only pill (POP). The over-the-counter preparation St John's Wort (Hypericum perforatum) also has properties as an hepatic enzyme inducer and should be treated as such. (Faculty of FP 2005). Newer anticonvulsants, such as sodium valproate and lamotrigine, do not have this effect. The potency of rifampicin's and rifabutin's induction of hepatic microsomal enzymes is such that alternative precautions should be taken even during very short, single-dose, concurrent use with oral contraceptives and for a month after the last dose (Faculty of FP 2005). Where other enzyme inducers are being used in the short term, additional contraceptive precautions are required during use and for 7 days afterwards. Where long-term use is required, alternative methods that are not susceptible to enzyme induction should be considered, such as Depo-Provera, Mirena and copper-containing IUDs. If this is not acceptable, a higher dose of COC can be prescribed to the equivalent of a 50 μg pill. A shortened pill-free interval (4 days), and 'tricycling' are recommended (see pp. 10–11); (NB this is off licence).

Antibiotics

Broad-spectrum antibiotics can affect metabolism of the COC by disturbing the gut flora and hence altering the enterohepatic circulation of oestrogen (Faculty of FP 2005), e.g. ampicillin, amoxicillin, tetracyclines. The evidence for this is mainly theoretical, but there are case reports of otherwise unexplained pill failures. As this is an effect on oestrogen levels, broad-spectrum antibiotics do not have a similar effect on the POP. It is also likely that the new non-oral oestrogen-progestogen methods, the EVRA patch and NuvaRing, are not affected by broad-spectrum antibiotics.

The British National Formulary (BNF) recommends additional precautions whilst taking the potentially interacting medicine and for at least 7 days after stopping it. If these 7 days run beyond the end of the packet, the new packet should be started immediately without a break.

Drug interactions where COC might affect the metabolism of another drug

Corticosteroids and other immunosuppressants

A number of studies have reported changes in prednisolone pharmacokinetics in COC users (Faculty of FP 2005). It has been suggested that lower doses of prednisolone are required to yield clinical efficiency in women taking COCs.

Cyclosporin

COCs have been reported as being responsible for increasing plasma concentrations of cyclosporins. *In vitro* studies have shown cyclosporin and COCs share metabolic pathways in the liver (Faculty of FP 2005).

Missing the pill-free interval

Although it cannot be denied that all research on the pill has been carried out in women having regular pill-free intervals (PFI), most women benefit from being able to skip them, at least occasionally, for holidays and so on. Indeed, for some women, the definite advantages of doing so easily outweigh the few theoretical disadvantages (Upadhyay 2005). Box 1.2 lists possible reasons for regularly omitting the PFI: tricycling, where the woman takes three packets in a row, followed by a break, is often a good compromise.

Box 1.2 Indications for regularly omitting the PFI

- Heavy or painful withdrawal bleeds
- Headaches, non-focal migraines or other symptoms which occur regularly in the PFI
- Women using enzyme-inducing drugs
- Previous unexplained pregnancy on the pill
- Absent withdrawal bleeds, if this causes the woman to be anxious about the risk of pregnancy
- Endometriosis
- At the woman's choice

Women who suffer with migraine during the PFI are a category who are often better served by a 20 μg pill, and also by tricycling (Upadhyay 2005). Obviously, one should first ascertain that they suffer from simple migraine, and not migraine with aura (see 'Migraine', above), which is an absolute contraindication to the combined pill.

A small study looking at older, high-dose pills showed that a potentially adverse effect of those pills on cholesterol was to some extent reversed during the pill-free week, and it was therefore suggested that the break might be useful in reducing the risks of cardiovascular disease. The newest pills do not have this effect on cholesterol, or any other significant metabolic effects. It seems less likely, therefore, that the breaks are beneficial from this point of view.

On the opposing side are the disadvantages of the pill-free week. They lead to pill omissions (women forget to restart), and therefore to pregnancies. They result in withdrawal bleeds, which can be a nuisance. Some women get side effects, such as headaches, or a kind of premenstrual syndrome during them.

Continuous pill taking is actually recommended in some gynaecological conditions, such as endometriosis, where bleeding is to be discouraged. It is also often recommended for epileptic women, since hormone fluctuations may encourage fits to occur. Tricycling is particularly recommended for women who get side effects related to the pill-free week, such as headaches, and for women who have heavy and/or painful withdrawal bleeds. In addition, it can be used in women who take hepatic enzyme-inducing drugs. The latter option is an off-licence use; current expert opinion and experience is that this is both safe and effective, although extensive data confirming this are not available.

However, it has long been recognized that many women, even without a specific medical reason, would prefer not to bleed unnecessarily 12 times a year. Such women have often chosen to tricycle their pill. Nevertheless, some women do find that if they don't have their 7-day break, they feel bloated and uncomfortable. Some of this may be psychological, but equally, the pill can cause slight water retention, and it may be that in some women it is enough to make them uncomfortable if they do not have a break (during which it presumably improves again). The majority of women do not have any problems skipping withdrawal bleeds occasionally.

Pill prescribing in polycystic ovarian syndrome (PCOS)

PCOS is a clinical syndrome characterized by hirsutism, obesity and oligo-amenorrhoea. The actual clinical features are variable both between patients and within individual patients over time. In the short term, PCOS is associated with dysfunctional uterine bleeding, which can be heavy, and infertility. Identified long-term risks are diabetes mellitus and endometrial carcinoma. A COC (including Dianette, see 'Acne', above) can therefore offer benefits to clients with acne, hirsutism and menstrual disturbance attributable to the condition. It would be usual to ensure that women with PCOS with a cycle longer than 8 weeks are treated to ensure a regular withdrawal bleed. The long-term effects on risk of diabetes, its complications or endometrial carcinoma are unknown but may be beneficial on the latter as the oestrogen predominance is reduced.

References and further reading

Belsey EM. (1988) The association between vaginal bleeding pattern and reasons for discontinuation of contraceptive use. *Contraception* **38**, 207–25.

Brill K, Muller C, Schnitker J, Albring M. (1991) The influence of different modern low-dose oral contraceptives on intermenstrual bleeding. *Adv Contraception* **7**(Suppl 2), 51–61.

Drug and Therapeutics Bulletin (1992) Starting oral contraceptives – which, when and how? Vol. 30, No.11.

Erkkola R, Hirvonen E, Luikku J, Lumme R, Mannikko H, Aydinlik S. (1990) Ovulation inhibitors containing cyproterone acetate or desogestrel in treatment of hyperandrogenic symptoms. *Acta Obstet Gynecol Scand* **69**, 61–5.

Faculty of Family Planning and Reproductive Health Care Clinical Effectiveness Unit. FFPRHC Guidance (April 2005) Drug interactions with hormonal contraception. *J Fam Plann Reprod Health Care* **31(2)** , 139-51.

Hillard PA. (1989) The patient's reaction to side-effects of oral contraceptives. *Am J Obstet Gynecol* **161**, 1412–15.

International Working Group on Enhancing Patient Compliance and Oral Contraceptive Efficacy (1993) Consensus statement. *Br J Fam Plann* **18**, 126–9.

Levrier M, Degrelle H, Bestaux Y, Bourry-Moreno M, Brun JP, Sailly F. (1989) Efficacy of oral contraceptives on acne. *Science Serv Int* 77–81.

Loudon NB, Kirkman RJE, Dewsbury JA. (1990) A double-blind comparison of the efficacy and acceptability of Femodene and Microgynon-30. *Eur J Obstet Gynecol Reprod Biol* **34**, 257–66.

MacGregor A. (2001) Hormonal contraception and migraine. *J Fam Plann Reprod Health Care* **27**(1), 49–52.

Mango D, Ricci S, Manna P, Miggiano GAD, Serra GB. (1996) Clinical and hormonal effects of ethinyloestradiol combined with gestodene and desogestrel in young women with acne vulgaris. *Contraception* **53**, 163–70.

Redmond GP, Olson WH, Lippman JS, Kafrissen ME, Jones TM, Jorizzo JL. (1997) Norgestimate and ethinyl estradiol in the treatment of acne vulgaris: a randomized, placebo-controlled trial. *Obstet Gynecol* **89**(4), 615–22.

Upadhyay, UD. (2005) *New contraceptive choices*. Population Reports, Series M, No. 19. Baltimore: Johns Hopkins Bloomberg School of Public Health, The INFO Project.

Van Vloten WA, van Haselen CW, van Zuuren EJ, Gerlinger C, Heithecker R. (2002) The effect of 2 combined oral contraceptives containing either drospirenone or cyproterone acetate on acne and seborrhoea. *Cutis* **69(4S)**, 2–15.

Walling M. (1998) Uncertainty remains over use of the pill. In: Oral contraceptives: results and interpretation of a GP survey on attitudes and prescribing habits. *Trends Interpreter* **January**.

Webb AMC. (1996) Do currently available combined oral contraceptives cause weight gain and other minor side effects? In: Hannaford PC, Webb AMC (eds), *Evidence-guided prescribing of the pill*. New York/London: Parthenon Press.

2 COMBINED ORAL CONTRACEPTIVES AND CANCER

As the majority of contraceptive users are healthy men and women, the safety of contraceptives is paramount. There is no more emotive aspect of safety than the effect of medication on malignancy. For non-hormonal contraceptives, there are no concerns of increased risk of malignancy and in fact condoms may actually one day be proven to be protective against cervical cancer. However, there are concerns about the effect of hormonal methods, not least because a number of cancers have been demonstrated to be sensitive to sex steroids through the expression of hormone receptors. The most studied hormonal method is the COC.

Demonstrating a link between COCs and cancer is complicated by two main factors:

- the length of time between exposure to carcinogen and being diagnosed as having cancer; and
- the fact that there are few women who have only used one method of contraception.

Most research into the link between cancer and the COC has been of an epidemiological nature. For the more common cancers, such as carcinoma of the breast and cervix, there are both cohort and case-controlled studies. However, even then it has been necessary to pool the results of multiple studies to achieve statistical significance. The need for very large studies to analyse the effect of the COC on cancer is one indication of the safety of the pill in this respect. Having said that, there are some important positive and negative effects that health-care professionals and users need to be aware of.

Primary liver cancer

Because of the very low incidence in the United Kingdom population, even large cohort studies have limited ability to investigate possible effects of COC use on liver disease. Published data on mortality trends are reassuring (Mant and Vessey 1995; Waetjen and Grimes 1996). Nine case-control studies were conducted in populations with low prevalence of hepatitis B and C, viral infection and chronic liver disease (which are major causes of liver cancer). In analyses where women with these factors were excluded, long-term use of COCs was associated with a small increase in the risk of hepatocellular carcinoma [International Agency for Research on Cancer (IARC) 1999]. The absolute risk (approximately 4 per million) is small and few long-term data are available on the more recent, low-dose formulations.

Hydatidiform mole/choriocarcinoma

In a large case series of women who have had choriocarcinoma (Newlands 1999) those women who received COC whilst their human chorionic gonadotropin (hCG) levels were still raised were significantly more likely subsequently to require chemotherapy than those whose hCG level had returned to normal before using exogenous hormones. Whether this is an effect of oestrogens or progestogens is unknown and it is recommended that all women being followed up for trophoblastic disease should avoid hormonal methods, including the COC, until the hCG levels (measured by a specialist laboratory) have returned to normal. Thereafter there are no restrictions on which contraceptive to use.

Ovarian cancer

An IARC review of the four cohort and 21 case-control studies that address the relationship between ovarian cancer and use of COCs found they consistently indicate a reduction in risk of about 50% for women who have used COCs for at least 5 years. Studies have shown a 40% reduction in the risk of developing ovarian cancer after only 3 years of pill taking. Further reductions in risk occur with longer use, and reach about 60% after 7 years. The effect appears to persist for 10–15 years after cessation of pill taking (IARC 1999). These data refer to the use of 50 μg COC pills. The effect is thought to be as a result of ovarian suppression, which also occurs with lower dose COCs. It is encouraging that although there are still relatively few studies, both high- and low-dose COCs appear to confer a similar level of protection (Deligeoroglou *et al.* 2003). Evidence is also mounting that COCs offer a similar level of protection against ovarian cancer for carriers of the BRCA1 and BRCA2 mutations (McGuire *et al.* 2004; Whittemore *et al.* 2004).

Endometrial cancer

An IARC review of the three cohort and 16 case-control studies that address the relationship between the use of COCs and the risk of endometrial cancer found that they consistently indicate a risk reduction of about 50% for women who have used COCs for at least 5 years. There is a reduced risk even after only one year of use, by a factor of 20%. At least 4 years of use are necessary to achieve the 50% reduction. As for ovarian cancer, this reduction seems to last for 10 years after use has ceased (IARC 1999, 2006; Cogliano *et al.* 2005).

Breast cancer

The risk of breast cancer in oral contraceptive users has been the topic of a number of pill scares in the last 15 years. An overview of 90% of the studies so far carried out (Collaborative Group on Hormonal Factors in Breast Cancer 1996) has been published and a recent IARC monograph has also reviewed the data (Cogliano *et al.* 2005; IARC 2006). It should be pointed out that this is not a new study in itself, simply a 'pulling together' of the data from other studies.

The review (Collaborative Group on Hormonal Factors in Breast Cancer 1996) suggests that there is a small increase in risk (relative risk 1.24) for women who are current users of oral contraceptives. This excess risk declines progressively after cessation of use, disappearing altogether after 10 years. There was no effect of duration of use, i.e. long-term users appeared to have the same risk as short-term users. In addition, there was no effect of pill dose, so use of high-dose pills carried the same risk as that of low-dose pills.

Another interesting finding was that the breast cancers diagnosed in pill users were clinically less advanced than those in never-users, and were less likely to have spread beyond the breast. This would suggest that mortality from breast cancer might actually be reduced in pill users (although this is not proven). The authors state that the lack of both a duration of use and a dose–response effect makes a causal association unlikely. There are two plausible explanations for these results, either or both of which may play a part.

First, it is possible that the pill accelerates the growth of tumours that were already present, thus making them clinically obvious earlier. A second possibility is that of surveillance bias, i.e. that women who take the pill are more 'breast aware' and are also more likely to be seeing doctors and nurses regularly, allowing the opportunity for advice and examinations. This would explain the earlier diagnosis in pill users compared with never-users, who may be less exposed to medical contact. The authors of the report are bemused by the fact that the earlier diagnosis also applies to ex-users of the pill: however, of course, once women have become 'breast aware', they do not suddenly become 'unaware' just because they have stopped taking the pill.

As always, an individual woman needs to assess the particular risks and benefits of the pill in relation to her own needs and medical history and these should be discussed with her.

Cervical cancer

There has, for many years, been a suggestion of an association between the COC pill and an increased risk of cervical intraepithelial neoplasia and invasive cervical cancer of both adeno and squamous varieties. However, because the most important risk factor is known to be sexually acquired infection with high-risk human papillomavirus (HPV) types, it has always been difficult to separate the possible effects of the COC from those of sexual behaviour.

The incidence of cervical carcinoma is declining in the UK. This is attributed to the cervical screening programme. In considering the effect of contraceptives on cervical cancer, the benefit of regular cervical screening should be borne in mind.

Smoking is a known co-factor that is more important than any effect that may be attributable to the COC. In developed countries, where many women smoke, smoking doubles the risk of cervical cancer. However, in developing countries, where few women smoke, other, concurrent sexually transmitted infections, which may be a marker for HPV acquisition, seem to be more important.

A number of studies (Cogliano *et al.* 2005; IARC 2006) have suggested an increase in cervical cancer in COC users; this effect appears to be duration dependent with no increase being demonstrated in users of less than 5 years.

A recent publication by Moreno *et al.* (2002) pooled the results of 10 cervical cancer case-control studies, mostly from developing countries. They restricted the analysis to women who tested positive for high-risk HPV types (both cases and controls). They found no increase in risk of cervical cancer for use of the pill of less than 5 years. For COC use of between 5 and 9 years, there appeared to be a trebling of risk, while use for more than 10 years appeared to increase the risk fourfold. However, these figures should be treated with caution, as there were only 12/14 controls, respectively, in these longer use categories. The increase in risk disappeared within 6 years of stopping the pill. Although this analysis does suggest that long-term users of the pill who are HPV positive may be at greater risk of cervical cancer, it does not prove that the pill actually causes cervical cancer.

Interestingly, they found that use of the pill was not associated with an increased risk of being HPV positive. Thus, the pill does not appear to enhance the chances of acquisition or persistence of HPV infection; if anything, the mechanism would be to promote progression to cancer after the HPV infection had become persistent. In the UK, at least 80% of women would have used the pill at some time in their lives: in these studies, only around a third of the women had ever used the pill and they may therefore not be representative of the general population. Recent studies in developed countries have not found a significant association with pill use (Deacon *et al.* 2000; Kjellberg *et al.* 2000; Coker *et al.* 2001; Moscicki *et al.* 2001).

Current advice is not to stop the COC when a woman is diagnosed as having cervical intraepithelial neoplasia unless there is another method that is more acceptable for the woman.

Colorectal cancer

Several studies have suggested an inverse association between current use of COCs and the risk of colorectal cancer (Fernandez *et al.* 2001; Levi *et al.* 2003). The relative risks for ever-use are around 0.8 (i.e. a 20% reduction), and when studies are combined, reach statistical significance (Fernandez *et al.* 2001). Duration of use does not appear to be associated with a decrease in risk. The mechanism for a protective effect is not understood, but may be related to changes in bile synthesis and secretion, inhibition of the growth of colon cancer cells and tumour suppressor genes (Fernandez *et al.* 2001).

Summary

The COC has a very good safety profile with regard to increased risks of malignancy and for some cancers the risks are reduced. The data on the COC and cancer risk have to be viewed in the overall context of benefits as well as risks of the pill. In addition to its high efficacy as a contraceptive, the pill has many health benefits. These range from reductions in menstrual cycle disorders (such as dysmenorrhoea, menorrhagia and premenstrual syndrome) to almost complete protection against benign breast disease and benign ovarian cysts. In addition, the method protects against pelvic inflammatory disease and ectopic pregnancy. The main issues are for older women using combined contraceptives and those with a family or personal history of breast cancer. As always, an individual woman needs to assess the particular risks and benefits of the pill in relation to her own needs and medical history.

References and further reading

Cogliano V, Grosse Y, Baan R *et al.* (2005) Carcinogenicity of combined oestrogen-progestagen contraceptives and menopausal treatment. *Lancet Oncol* **6**, 552–3.

Coker AL, Sanders LC, Bond SM, Gerasimova T, Pirisi L. (2001) Hormonal and barrier methods of contraception, oncogenic human papillomaviruses and cervical squamous intraepithelial lesion development. *J Women's Health Gender-based Med* **10**(5), 44.

Collaborative Group on Hormonal Factors in Breast Cancer (1996) Breast cancer and hormonal contraceptives: collaborative reanalysis of individual data on 53 297 women with breast cancer and 100 239 women without breast cancer from 54 epidemiological studies. *Lancet* **347**, 1713–27.

Deacon JM, Evans CD, Yule R, Desai M, Binns W, Taylor C, Peto J. (2000) Sexual behaviour and smoking as determinants of cervical HPV infection and of CIN 3 among those infected: a case-control study nested within the Manchester cohort. *Br J Cancer* **88**(11), 1565–72.

Deligeoroglou E, Michailidis E, Creatsas G. (2003) Oral contraceptives and reproductive system cancer. *Ann N Y Acad Sci.* **997**,199–208.

Fernandez E, La Vecchia C, Balducci A, Chatenoud L, Franceschi S, Negri E. (2001) Oral contraceptives and colorectal cancer risk: a meta-analysis. *Br J Cancer* **84**, 722–7.

International Agency for Research on Cancer (1999) Monographs on the evaluation of carcinogenic risks to humans. Volume 72. *Hormonal contraception and post-menopausal hormonal therapy.* Lyons: WHO IARC.

International Agency for Research on Cancer (2006) IARC monographs on the evaluation of carcinogenic risks to humans, volume 91, combined estrogen-progestogen contraceptives and combined estrogen-progestogen menopausal therapy. Lyons: IARC (in press).

Kjellberg L, Hallmans G, Ahren AM *et al.* (2000) Smoking, diet, pregnancy and oral contraceptive use as risk factors for cervical intra-epithelial neoplasia in relation to human papillomavirus infection. *Br J Cancer* **82**(7), 1332–8.

Levi F, Pasche C, Lucchini F, La Vecchia C. (2003) Oral contraceptives and colorectal cancer. *Dig Liver Dis* **35**(2), 85–7.

McGuire V, Felberg A, Mills M, Ostrow KL, DiCioccio R, John EM, West DW, Whittemore AS. (2004) Relation of contraceptive and reproductive history to ovarian cancer risk in carriers and noncarriers of BRCA1 gene mutations. *Am J Epidemiol* **160**, 613–18.

Mant JW, Vessey MP. (1995) Trends in mortality from primary liver cancer in England and Wales 1975–92: influence of oral contraceptives. *Br J Cancer* **72**(3), 800–3.

Moreno V, Bosch FX, Munoz N *et al.* (2002) Effect of oral contraceptives on risk of cervical cancer in women with human papillomavirus infection: the IARC multicentric case-control study. *Lancet* **359**, 1085–92.

Moscicki AB, Hills N, Shiboski S *et al.* (2001) Risks for incident human papillomavirus infection and low grade squamous intraepithelial lesion development in young females. *J Am Med Assoc* **285**, 2995–3002.

Newlands ES. (1999) Human chorionic gonadotrophin monitoring, hormonal contraception and pregnancy in patients with trophoblastic disease. *Hormones and cancer.* London: RCOG Hormone Study Group.

Waetjen LE, Grimes DA. (1996) Oral contraceptives and primary liver cancer: temporal trends in three countries. *Obstet Gynecol* **88**(6), 945–9.

Whittemore AS, Balise RR, Pharoah PD *et al.* (2004) Oral contraceptive use and ovarian cancer risk among carriers of BRCA1 or BRCA2 mutations. *Br J Cancer* doi:10.1038/sj.bjc.6602239

3 THE EFFECT OF DEPO-PROVERA ON BONE DENSITY AND ARTERIAL DISEASE

Depo-Provera (depomedroxyprogesterone acetate) is a safe, effective and very acceptable method of contraception for many women, especially younger women who find remembering to take oral contraceptives difficult. In recent years there have been two main areas of controversy regarding the safety of Depo-Provera, the effect on bone density and on arterial disease.

Bone density

There has been much discussion in the last 10 years about the possibility of a reduction in bone density with long-term Depo-Provera use, due to ovarian suppression. This was first raised in 1991 when Cundy *et al.* reported a cross-sectional study of 30 amenorrhoeic long-term users of Depo-Provera. Long-term (more than 5 years) Depo-Provera users had a 7% lower bone mass compared to premenopausal controls. However, there were a number of problems with the study design (in particular, matching of cases and controls) and therefore it contributed little other than by drawing attention to this area. Cundy has since published a larger study (Cundy *et al.* 1998), with similar findings, but he has again used volunteers and therefore bias may still account for his results. It is also unlikely that the difference in bone mineral density (BMD) observed is of any clinical significance.

A similar sized study, using consecutive clinic attendees (with 91% compliance) from the UK has not confirmed Cundy's findings (Gbolade *et al.* 1998) and is therefore reassuring. Although the majority of Depo-Provera users had low oestradiol levels, this bore no correlation with their bone densities (see below). A major problem in the studies published so far is that women who choose or are advised to use Depo-Provera appear to be highly likely to have risk factors for osteoporosis, such as smoking and low socioeconomic status. This makes comparisons with users of other methods very difficult, and it is quite possible that the observed differences in bone density are due to these risk factors, and not the Depo-Provera itself.

Studies have shown conflicting results, but, in summary, any change in BMD secondary to Depo-Provera use, if any, is small, non-progressive and not related to duration of use. Of greater concern is the effect of long-term use of Depo-Provera on the bone density of adolescents (Cromer *et al.* 2005; Cromer 2005; Scholes *et al.* 2004, 2005). Most of the bone mass in the spine and hip is accumulated by the age of 18 years. Since attainment of peak bone density appears to be the single most useful measure to prevent osteoporosis and fractures in later life, it would seem prudent to avoid any drugs that would prevent attainment of peak bone density during adolescence. The CSM has recently issued advice regarding use of Depo-Provera (MHRA 2004), which states:

- In adolescents, Depo-Provera may be used as first-line contraception but **only** after other methods have been discussed with the patient and considered to be unsuitable or unacceptable;
- In women of all ages, careful re-evaluation of the risks and benefits of treatment should be carried out in those who wish to continue use for more than 2 years;
- In women with significant lifestyle and/or medical risk factors for osteoporosis, other methods of contraception should be considered.

The MHRA advice does not specify what form the 2-year re-evaluation should take. In particular, there is no suggestion that this re-evaluation need include bone density measurement. The Faculty of Family Planning has stated that on the basis of current evidence available, no laboratory tests or imaging procedures are required as a routine. In October 2005 NICE published its guidance on Long Acting Reversible Contraceptives, which included DMPA; this reviewed the current evidence and, whilst acknowledging the MHRA guidance, is supportive to the long-term use of DMPA.

Depo-Provera acts on the hypothalamic–pituitary–ovarian axis and reduces peak levels of luteinizing hormone (LH) and follicle-stimulating hormone (FSH). This leads to an associated reduction in the cyclical variation of oestradiol, with levels generally being similar to those found in the early follicular phase of ovulatory cycles.

It has been suggested that measurement of serum oestradiol should be carried out in long-term users. However, there are no studies showing a

Box 3.1 Risk factors for osteoporosis

- Smoking
- Ethnicity
- Family history
- Low levels of exercise
- Low socioeconomic status

linear relationship between oestradiol levels and BMD: on the contrary, there are two studies which have shown no correlation. Therefore, this test is not useful and is not recommended in this situation.

Depo-Provera users may, as individuals, be at risk of osteoporosis because of their other characteristics (see Box 3.1) and clearly if a woman is suspected of having osteopenia or osteoporosis, measurement of BMD is indicated. Unfortunately, bone scans are often difficult to access. It therefore may be appropriate to assess long-term users of Depo-Provera on the basis of their other, known risk factors for osteoporosis, rather than their use of Depo-Provera. Long-term users are generally very happy with their method and not keen to change: in addition, the obvious bone-conserving option of the combined pill may be contraindicated if they are smokers over the age of 35. Thus, if a woman is approaching the menopause, is a smoker and perhaps has other risk factors, one could (either following confirmation with a bone density scan or just pragmatically) suggest that she starts hormone replacement therapy (HRT) early (as do many women not on Depo-Provera). Protection from endometrial cancer has been shown in Depo users and although outside the product licence, it is then possible to use Depo-Provera as the progestogen part of the HRT, while adding oestradiol in whatever form the woman prefers.

Arterial disease

There has also been debate regarding arterial disease risk in long-term users, particularly as a result of a study in which 12 women used Depo-Provera for at least one year and were compared to nine controls (Sorensen *et al.* 2002). Using magnetic resonance imaging, the researchers evaluated arterial function by monitoring changes in the brachial artery. The results suggested that arterial function might be slightly impaired in the Depo users. The small size of the study, the recency of the technique, and the focus on a microscopic, non-clinical end point, should make us wary of drawing conclusions or changing our practice. In addition, an epidemiological study looking at arterial disease in Depo-Provera users has found no increase in risk (WHO Collaborative Study of Cardiovascular Disease and Steroid Hormone Contraception 1998). It has been known for many years that Depo-Provera may slightly lower HDL levels: in view of this, it has generally been suggested that for women with strong risk factors for arterial disease, Depo-Provera may not be the best choice, especially as there are lower-dose progestogen-only methods available.

References and further reading

Cromer BA. (2005) In favor of continued use of depot medroxyprogesterone acetate (DMPA, Depo-Provera) in adolescents. *J Pediatr Adolesc Gynecol* **18**(3), 183–7.

Cromer BA, Lazebnik R, Rome E, Stager M, Bonny A, Ziegler J, Debanne SM. (2005) Double-blinded randomized controlled trial of estrogen supplementation in adolescent girls who receive depot medroxyprogesterone acetate for contraception. *Am J Obstet Gynecol* **192**(1), 42–7.

Cundy T, Evans M, Roberts H, Wattie D, Ames R, Reid I. (1991) Bone density in women receiving depot medroxyprogesterone acetate for contraception. *Br Med J* **303**, 13–16.

Cundy T, Cornish J, Roberts H, Elder H, Reid I. (1998) Spinal bone density in women using depot medroxyprogesterone contraception. *Obstet Gynecol* **92**, 569–73.

Gbolade BA. (2002) Depo-Provera and bone density. *J Fam Plann Reprod Health Care* **28**(1), 7–11.

Gbolade B, Ellis S, Murby B, Randall S, Kirkman R. (1998) Bone density in long-term users of depot medroxyprogesterone acetate *Br J Obstet Gynaecol* **105**, 790–4.

MHRA statement on Depo Provera, 19.11.04 http://medicines.mhra.gov.uk/ourwork/monitorsafequalmed/safetymessages/urgent.htm

Scholes D, LaCroix AZ, Ichikawa LE, Barlow WE, Ott SM. (2004) The association between depot medroxyprogesterone acetate contraception and bone mineral density in adolescent women. *Contraception* **69**, 99–104.

Scholes D, LaCroix AZ, Ichikawa LE, Barlow WE, Ott SM. (2005) Change in bone mineral density among adolescent women using and discontinuing depot medroxyprogesterone acetate contraception. *Arch Pediatr Adolesc Med* **159**(2), 139–44.

Sorensen MB, Collins P, Ong PJ *et al.* (2002) Long-term use of contraceptive depot medroxyprogesterone acetate in young women impairs arterial endothelial function assessed by cardiovascular magnetic resonance. *Circulation* **106**, 1646–51.
WHO Collaborative Study of Cardiovascular Disease and Steroid Hormone Contraception (1998) Cardiovascular disease and use of oral and injectable progestogen-only contraceptives and combined injectable contraceptives. *Contraception* **57**, 315–24.

4 INTRAUTERINE DEVICES (IUDS)

Intrauterine devices and infection

For many years the poorly understood link between 'infection' and IUDs has been a major barrier to their use. The perception that IUDs are the primary cause of pelvic inflammatory disease (PID) when it occurs anytime after insertion is not uncommon both amongst patients and the medical and nursing professions and is incorrect. This almost certainly denies many women a safe, highly effective, long-term method of contraception. IUDs are also cheap, some costing less than £10, and have a proven 10-year life span.

Our current understanding of the relationship between intrauterine devices and infection needs to consider the link with three conditions: PID, bacterial vaginosis (BV) and actinomycosis/*Actinomyces*-like organisms (ALOs) on cervical cytology.

Pelvic inflammatory disease (PID)

Concerns over the risk of PID have restricted the use of IUDs because of the possibility of subsequent tubal factor infertility. This concern was often regarded as being greatest for nulliparous women. Whilst it is true that there is a small increase in the risk of PID attributable to IUD insertion, this is exceedingly low, at approximately 0.1%. Significant increased risk is, however, limited to situations when a cervical sexually transmitted infection (STI) is also present: in this situation the risk of post-insertion PID has been estimated to be about 5%. It has also been demonstrated that the risk is increased only for the first 20 days after insertion; after this time the risk is the same as the background risk. A single episode of PID results in a 9% chance of subsequent tubal infertility and an increase in the risk of ectopic pregnancy. Whilst the attributable risk is low in women without an STI, there is still a small risk of developing PID that is not present or may be reduced with other methods of contraception. This is acceptable to many women and if STI has been excluded, the decision to use an IUD should be that of the user, including young nulliparous women. These risks can be compared to the risk of post-abortal PID, which is between 5 and 15%; again this is STI dependent.

In studies of copper IUDs, the type of device does not alter the risk of developing PID. The Mirena intrauterine system (IUS) has been demonstrated not to result in an increased risk of PID and, although conflicting evidence exists, some studies have demonstrated the IUS to have a lower than background risk beyond 20 days. This is probably due to a progestogenic protective effect against ascending infection by altering the cervical mucous.

There are few studies of long-term fertility after use of intrauterine contraception but the results of these conflict with our understanding of the known risks of PID and are poorly controlled; further work is expected in this area.

Treatment of PID

Treatment of PID in an IUD user should be as for a non-IUD user. Appropriate swabs should be taken to exclude STI and antimicrobial therapy prescribed against chlamydia, anaerobes and, if relevant, gonorrhoea. Partner notification is recommended. Alternative methods may be discussed but the device should not be removed if it is that woman's choice of contraception, unless her condition does not respond to treatment and it is certain that PID is the cause of her symptoms. It is not recommended to reinsert an IUD until she is clinically cured and tests for STI are negative (Faculty of FP 2004)

Prevention of post-insertion PID

Women who do not have an STI are at very low risk of developing post-insertion PID and subsequent infertility or ectopic pregnancy, irrespective of age and parity. In the absence of other contraindicating factors, the discriminating factor in whether to fit an IUD is therefore the risk for an STI and not age or parity. It is therefore recommended that a sexual history should be taken to assess risk for STI, to offer all women tests for STI and to ensure the results are back and negative before inserting the IUD. For women who have had a recent STI, having excluded treatment failure and re-infection, it is not unreasonable to insert an IUD if that is going to be the most acceptable and best method for her.

Unlike post-abortal PID, there is no evidence that prophylactic antibiotics reduce the risk of PID. However, it is usual to offer treatment against chlamydia and anaerobes to women having an emergency IUD if there is a potential STI risk.

Bacterial vaginosis

BV is a common cause of vaginal discharge with an estimated prevalence of up to 20% in some populations. Many women are asymptomatic. This condition, which is not sexually transmitted, is associated with an increased malodorous vaginal discharge, commonly described as being fishy in smell. There is no single and universally accepted test for BV. In the UK, Gram staining is used widely in genitourinary medicine (GUM) clinics (BASHH Guidelines) but this is not practical for most clinical situations where BV presents and modified Amsel's criteria are often used (Box 4.1).

Box 4.1 Diagnosis of BV – Amsel's criteria

Three of four criteria are required to make a diagnosis of BV:

- presence of characteristic homogeneous discharge;
- vaginal fluid pH >4.5;
- positive amine test;
- Gram stained smear of vaginal discharge demonstrating 'clue' cells.

Modified Amsel's criteria utilize only the first two conditions in Box 4.1 with a high vaginal swab (HVS) being sent for Gram staining if the local laboratory does this.

A number of studies have demonstrated a link between BV and IUD use; however, other well conducted studies have not. There are also anecdotal reports of women with persistent or recurrent symptomatic BV being 'cured' by removal of the IUD. The reasons for the difference in the studies may be due to poor control for other confounding factors, such as smoking, condom use and douching and the use of different diagnostic methods. There may therefore be a link between BV and IUD use, but it must be remembered that BV is a common condition that commonly recurs and, if a woman wishes to use an IUD as her method, its removal should only be recommended as a last resort.

IUD use with *Actinomyces*-like organisms on cervical cytology

In the 1970s it was recognized that amongst women using IUDs there was an increase in the chance of having a cervical smear reported as showing *Actinomyces*-like organisms (ALOs). Pelvic actinomycosis is a very rare condition; being a chronic granulomatous pelvic infection, it is, however, quite debilitating and can be difficult to treat. Some women diagnosed as having pelvic actinomycosis have been IUD users.

Cervical smears are not designed to identify cervical colonization with *Actinomyces israelii.* ALOs are, however, seen on smears of women using IUDs: whilst some of these findings are actually due to other non-pathogenic organisms, it cannot be ruled out that they represent *Actinomyces israelii.* The significance of the findings with regard to actual risk of developing pelvic actinomycosis is controversial, but there is general agreement that not only should the woman be informed of the findings, but also of the possible (very small) risk and the management options. The management options are also controversial, with many favouring exclusion of any evidence of pelvic disease alone.

If the patient is symptomatic of pelvic infection or has clinical signs that are consistent with pelvic actinomycosis (pelvic tenderness or mass), further gynaecological investigation is warranted. An IUD that is removed from a symptomatic woman should have the threads cut off and be sent in a dry sterile container for culture of *Actinomyces.*

Asymptomatic women with an incidental finding of ALOs on cervical cytology should have a clinical examination to exclude any findings consistent with pelvic actinomycosis. If the examination is normal there are two options. The first, and most common line of management, is to counsel the patient about the small possibility of developing a problem and advise her to report any relevant symptoms and to review her 6-monthly. The other option is to remove and replace the IUD after STI risk assessment. The latter option is based on a study demonstrating that 3 months after replacement of the IUD, the cervical smear did not show persistence of ALOs. However, there has been no long-term follow-up of either management option and the risk of removal and replacement must be considered against the almost negligible risk of pelvic actinomycosis and any concern of the patient. Whatever management option is taken, cervical smears should not be repeated any more frequently than as indicated by the NHS cervical screening programme.

Past history of ectopic pregnancy: IUD or not?

It is now well recognized that prevention of fertilization is the main mechanism of action of IUDs and the progestogen-only Mirena IUS. A reduction in ectopic pregnancy rate has been demonstrated for both IUDs containing more than 380 mm^2 of copper and the IUS. However, although failure is very rare with these devices, when it does occur there is a one in 20 risk of ectopic pregnancy (NICE LARC Guideline 2005). This compares with a one in 100 risk in women not using contraception. However, the absolute risk is lower in women using an IUD or IUS because the chance of pregnancy is so much less. Women who have had a previous ectopic pregnancy have at least a one in 20 risk of recurrence if not using any method of contraception. A high dose IUD or IUS will significantly reduce this risk for the reasons just described. Women with a history of a previous ectopic pregnancy can therefore use these, if ovulation-inhibiting methods are not acceptable.

Which IUD?

The most effective IUDs contain at least 380 mm^2 of copper and have banded copper on the arms. Furthermore, the majority of the complications associated with IUD use, such as perforation, infection or expulsion, are related temporally or directly to the insertion process. It therefore seems logical to minimize the frequency of reinsertions in women using IUDs long term by using devices with an established effective lifespan of greater than 5 years (NICE LARC 2005). Currently licensed IUDs fulfilling these criteria are the 'T Safe Cu380A' and the 'TT380 Slimline', which, from the point of view of effectiveness and lifespan, are the IUDs of choice.

References and further reading

Cayley J, Fotherby K, Guillebaud J *et al.* (1998) Recommendations for clinical practice: actinomyces like organisms and intrauterine contraception. *Br J Fam Plann* **23**(4), 137–8.

Dennis J, Hampton N. (2002) IUDs: which device? Review. *J Fam Plann Reprod Health Care* **28**(2), 61–8.

Faculty of Family Planning and Reproductive Health Care Clinical Effectiveness Unit. FFPRHC Guidance (January 2004) The copper intrauterine device as long-term contraception. *J Family Plann Reprod Health Care* **30**(1), 29–42.

NICE LARC Guidance (2005) *Long-acting reversible contraception: the effective and appropriate use of long-acting reversible contraception.* London: National Institute for Health and Clinical Excellence.

UK national guidelines for the management of pelvic inflammatory disease. (2002) www.BASHH.org.uk.

UK national guidelines for the management of bacterial vaginosis. (2002) www.bashh.org.uk.

5 CONDOMS

Male condoms are an effective method of contraception, with the additional benefit of protection against sexually transmitted infections. This benefit is best against the bacterial infections gonorrhoea, chlamydia or trichomoniasis. However, there is also significant protection against the blood-borne viruses HIV and hepatitis B and C. Conditions that may affect the vulva and shaft of penis, such as warts and herpes, are less well prevented. Contraceptive failure rates of condoms are quoted as between two and 12 per 100 woman-years, depending on how consistent and correct their use is. All users of condoms should be aware of how to recognize condom failure and the availability of emergency contraception. Given the increasing failure rate of oral emergency contraception with time since intercourse, there is a strong argument to give emergency contraception to condom users in advance of its request, especially if the user is going abroad on holiday. This practice is known as advance prescribing.

There is some evidence that regular use of condoms leads to a lower risk of cervical intraepithelial neoplasia (Bleeker *et al.* 2005). For many women, particularly those who are young and who may not yet be in permanent monogamous relationships, the use of condoms is generally recommended as additional protection in conjunction with hormonal or intrauterine methods of contraception – the so-called 'double Dutch' method, providing effective contraception combined with protection against sexually transmitted diseases.

The use of male barriers to protect against sexually transmitted diseases was first documented about 3000 years ago; it is only within the last 1000 years that their use as contraceptives was recognized. Despite this long history, the condom is still undergoing development. Some of these developments could be regarded as being somewhat frivolous, such as flavoured, ribbed or coloured condoms. However, it is recognized that these developments, as well as contemporary branding and design of packaging, makes condoms more acceptable to some users, especially the young. All these developments are really about making a generally unacceptable method of protection against unplanned pregnancy and STIs more acceptable to the target users, which can only be a good thing.

Amongst the most commonly reported negative aspects of condom use are:

- interruption to lovemaking;
- lack of sensitivity;
- contact dermatitis and allergy.

Various attempts have been made to improve these issues, such as the polyurethane female condom Femidom and the latex Durex Gold condom, which is said to be easier to apply and is packed such that it is easier to put it on the right way round. Another more innovative product is the eZ•on® condom (Figure 5.1), made of elastomeric polyurethane, with a special soft flange, allowing it to be pulled on like a sock. It has no inside or outside, so it can be pulled on in either direction. The flange grips the base of the penis, but otherwise allows free movement of the penis within the condom. Because this should improve sensation for the man, they have been able to make the plastic particularly strong, so this type of condom should not break easily. Early trials suggest that it may be popular with both men and women (Gardner *et al.* 1999).

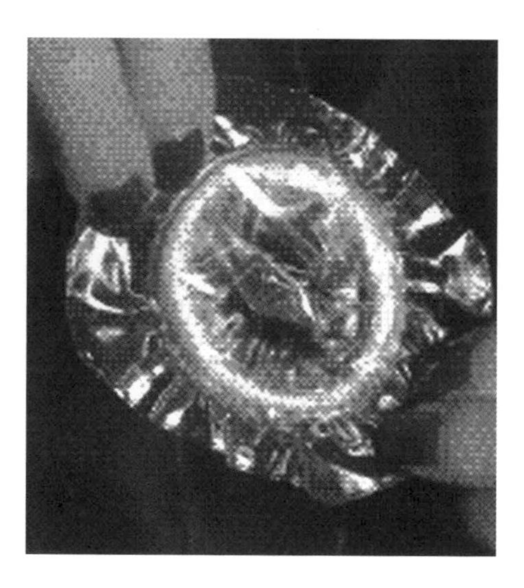

Figure 5.1 eZ•on® bidirectional polyurethane male condom. Photograph courtesy of Mayer Laboratories Inc., Oakland, CA 94606, USA.

Sensitivity

As a general rule, thinner condoms are regarded as providing greater sensitivity for the wearer but this is at the expense of strength. Whilst thicker condoms should be recommended for anal intercourse, any condom is better than no condom and the use of additional non-spermicidal lubricant is strongly advised. Sensation varies between individuals and it is hard to be dogmatic on whether well-fitting condoms offer greater or lesser sensitivity than loose-fitting ones. A wide range of sizes and shapes are available and people having problems with one type should be encouraged to try others before giving up on condoms altogether!

Contact dermatitis and allergy

After condom use, some men and women experience symptoms of allergy to latex or dermatitis, secondary to spermicidal lubricant. Common symptoms are local pruritus or soreness and burning; these occur during or after coitus and are usually short lived but can last for up to a week. Clinical examination is often normal, although erythema and occasionally swelling and epithelial disruption can occur. Douching or the use of topical vaginal hygiene products may appear to relieve symptoms but are not the solution to the problem. Caution should be taken not to misdiagnose these conditions as genital herpes or infective vulvovaginitis. In perimenopausal women, hypo-oestrogenic genital atrophy may lead to dryness, superficial dyspareunia and postcoital bleeding, which may be exacerbated by latex allergy or chemical dermatitis.

In the UK, most condoms are now lubricated with non-spermicidal lubricant, but those that do have a spermicidal lubricant contain nonoxinol 9 as the active ingredient. Nonoxinol 9 is also available as vaginal gels, creams, foams and pessaries for use either in association with vaginal diaphragms and cervical caps, or as a contraceptive in its own right. The latter are regarded to have an unacceptably low efficacy in younger women but may be acceptable in older women.

Spermicides such as nonoxinol 9 and other related compounds have been shown to have microbicidal activity but offer no protection against chlamydia, gonorrhoea or trichomoniasis. More importantly, when spermicide-containing sponges were used frequently by women at high risk for HIV, there was an increased rate of transmission of HIV secondary to epithelial disruption. This effect was dose related. It is unlikely that the small amount of nonoxinol 9 on some condoms, or used by most women using vaginal diaphragms, has a similar effect or that there are any adverse effects in women at low risk of HIV apart from the risk of local dermatitis. However, there is no evidence that spermicidally lubricated condoms offer greater protection against pregnancy than those using silicone lubricants. There is thus no evidence to support the use of spermicidally lubricated rather than non-spermicidally lubricated condoms (WHO/CONRAD 2001). There is considerable interest in finding new spermicides. Chlorhexidine and other vaginally applied substances are being researched for efficacy both for their contraceptive effect and also for protection against HIV infection. Gossypol, the Chinese drug derived from cottonseed oil, is also being tested as a vaginal contraceptive gel.

Until a few years ago, only latex rubber condoms were available in the UK. These have the disadvantage of latex allergy and susceptibility to chemical damage. Damage to condoms can occur with everyday hygiene products (see Table 5.1). Polyurethane condoms have been developed, such as Avanti, Femidom and eZ•on®, to overcome some of the problems associated with latex condoms. Polyurethane condoms

Table 5.1 Products known to weaken latex condoms*

Oil-based products	Topical medicinal products
Petroleum jelly (KY jelly is water-based and therefore safe)	Gyno-Daktarin cream and pessaries
E45 cream	Gyno-Pevaryl cream and pessaries (but Pevaryl is safe)
Skin lotions	Nystan cream (but pessaries are safe)
Suntan lotions	Monistat cream
Face creams	Ecostatin cream and pessaries
Edible creams	Sultrin cream
Butter or margarine	Oestrogen creams, such as those used in hormone replacement therapy (e.g. Premarin, Ortho-Dienoestrol)
Oil of any kind	Cyclogest (sometimes used for treatment of premenstrual syndrome)

*Individual products named are generally recognized as potentially weakening latex condoms. Classes of products may include preparations that do not, but good data are not available.

also have a longer shelf life than latex condoms. However, latex condoms have lower breakage, and lower slippage rates in normal use than polyurethane condoms.

Products known to be safe for use with condoms or diaphragms are shown in Box 5.1.

Box 5.1 Safe for use with condoms or diaphragms

- KY Jelly (or other water-based lubricants)
- Spermicidal creams and pessaries
- Senselle (now called Sensilube)
- Replens
- Aci-jel
- Betadine
- Canesten cream and pessaries
- Pevaryl cream
- Glycerine

References and further reading

Bleeker MC, Berkhof J, Hogewoning CJ *et al.* (2005) HPV type concordance in sexual couples determines the effect of condoms on regression of flat penile lesions. *Br J Cancer* **92**(8), 1388–92.

Gardner R, Blackburn RD, Upadhyay UD. (1999) *Closing the condom gap.* Population Reports, Series H, No. 9., Population Information Program. Baltimore: Johns Hopkins University School of Public Health.

WHO/CONRAD (2001) Nonoxynol-9. Technical Consultation, October 2001.

6 RECENT AND FUTURE CONTRACEPTIVE METHODS

Yasmin

Yasmin is a new combined oral contraceptive (COC) containing 30 µg ethinylestradiol plus 3 mg drospirenone. Drospirenone is a progestogen that closely resembles natural progesterone and has both anti-mineralocorticoid and anti-androgenic effects.

The production of renin by the kidneys leads to the release of angiotensin. This hormone stimulates the adrenal glands to produce aldosterone, which makes the kidney tubules reabsorb salt and water (this is known as the RAAS system). Normally, this is triggered by, for example, a fall in blood pressure. Oestrogen has a tendency to stimulate the production of renin, which triggers the RAAS cascade and results in salt and water retention. This is the reason for water retention and bloating that some women experience on the combined pill, and can also contribute to an increase in breast size and breast tenderness. Natural progesterone tends to block the effects of aldosterone by competing for the same receptors. By doing this, it effectively reduces water and salt retention.

This anti-mineralocorticoid action is an important difference between natural progesterone and the synthetic progestogens, apart from drospirenone. Drospirenone has been shown to have anti-mineralocorticoid activity, which is very similar to that of natural progesterone.

In a randomized, open-label study, Yasmin provided excellent contraceptive protection. A total of 9563 treatment cycles with Yasmin and 9498 with Marvelon were available for analysis and during these cycles six women became pregnant, three in each group (Foidart *et al.* 2000). This gives an uncorrected Pearl Index of 0.41 in both groups. However, in each case there was evidence of either pill-taking errors or other user factors that would have compromised efficacy. Both preparations provided good cycle control and their influence on haemostatic parameters, lipids and carbohydrate metabolism was clinically not significant.

A statistically significant difference was found in body weight changes between the Yasmin and the Marvelon group. While there was an increase in mean body weight in the Marvelon group from cycle 5 onwards, the mean body weight per cycle of the Yasmin group was slightly below the baseline value throughout the study. Similar results were seen in a larger, but shorter-term randomized study (Huber *et al.* 2000), again comparing Yasmin with Marvelon, and in a small randomized study comparing Yasmin with Microgynon (Oelkers *et al.* 1995). These data refer to mean body weight, not individual body weight, and there is no evidence that there is a long-term reduction in mean body weight below the baseline in Yasmin users.

Another study showed a significant improvement in premenstrual syndrome symptoms for women on Yasmin (Parsey and Pong 2000). Statistical significance comparing pre- and post-treatment was obtained for mood, water retention and increased appetite.

The randomized trials (Foidart *et al.* 2000; Huber *et al.* 2000) comparing Yasmin with Marvelon showed that both pills were equally beneficial for acne. A randomized, double-blind trial of 125 women has compared Yasmin (82 women) with Dianette (43 women). This showed that Yasmin was as effective as Dianette for women with mild to moderate acne (Van Vloten *et al.* 2002) There are no Yasmin data on hirsutism at the moment.

With regard to venous thromboembolism (VTE) risk, there are an estimated 1 million woman-years of use. The spontaneously observed reporting rate of VTE is currently approximately 6 per 100 000 woman-years of use. Recent data (the EURAS study) suggest no difference in VTE rates between second/third-generation pills, or Yasmin (Heinemann and Dinger 2004). The same study suggests that all VTE rates (including those in pregnancy) are higher than previously thought: those for the COC are between 60 and 73 per 100 000 women-years, while the risk in pregnancy reaches as high as 800 per 100 000 women-years (see Chapter 9)

Cerazette

Cerazette is a new progestogen-only pill (POP; 75 µg desogestrel daily) designed to inhibit ovulation. Whilst existing POPs can cause disrupted ovulation in up to 50% of users, they also rely heavily on cervical mucus and endometrial effects. A study comparing Cerazette with Microval showed that only 1.7% of cycles were ovulatory in Cerazette users, compared to 40% in Microval users (Rice *et al.* 1999). In a randomized trial of Cerazette versus Microval, the Pearl Index was 0.17 (method failure) and 0.5 (user failure) for Cerazette compared with 1.4 (method failure) and 1.9 (user failure) for Microval in non-breast-feeding women (Korver *et al.* 1998). Although the bleeding pattern in Cerazette users is more variable than with Microval, there is a greater tendency towards infrequent bleeding and amenorrhoea by the end of the first year. It would appear reasonable, in view of the ovulation inhibition, that there could be a 12-hour pill-taking safety margin rather than the three hours normally advised for conventional POPs (Korver *et al.* 2005). In June 2004 the Cerazette licence was revised to allow a 12-hour window for missed pills. Removal of the 'fear of forgetting' should make it a much more attractive option for many women.

Doubling the daily dose of conventional POPs has been suggested as a policy in women who weigh more than 70 kg, and indeed is mentioned in the Family Planning Association (FPA) leaflet on POPs. There is, however, no evidence relating to the POP itself to suggest that there is indeed an increased failure rate in overweight women (Vessey 2001). What evidence exists relates to a progestogen-only vaginal ring (which was not marketed) and an early version of Norplant; for both these devices, the failure rate was two to four times higher in women weighing 70 kg or more. However, in the case of Norplant, a change in the density of the polymer was enough to deal with the problem, so the marketed version was not significantly affected by weight. The efficacy of Implanon also does not appear to be affected by weight. Thus, there seems little justification for such a policy for the POP. However, in the case of young women using conventional POPs, it might be reasonable to err on the side of caution in view of the already higher failure rate. It would appear that this will not be necessary with Cerazette, since blood levels, as with Implanon, are high enough to withstand any effect of increased weight.

Emergency contraception update

Emergency contraception has become simpler. Recent evidence suggests that the efficacy of Levonelle is the same regardless of whether the pills are taken 12 hours apart, or both together (von Hertzen 2002; Webb 2003). Clearly, taking two pills at once (i.e. 1.5 mg levonorgestrel) is much simpler and is likely to improve compliance.

This stat dose regimen is licensed and new packaging has been available since January 2004. A single tablet version is now available both through pharmacies (Levonelle One Step, November 2004) and on prescription (Levonelle 1500, November 2005). When discussing emergency contraception, the role of the IUD, which is a more effective emergency contraceptive, should always be borne in mind. Whilst this will not be the method of choice for most women, current national guidance recommends that all women requesting emergency contraception should be fully counselled regarding the failure rates of oral and intrauterine emergency contraception to allow them to make an informed choice, even if they attend within 72 hours of unprotected intercourse (Faculty of FP 2004).

New non-oral routes of administration

Combined contraceptives offer highly effective and reversible protection against pregnancy in combination with good cycle control, but rely on daily intake of tablets. Contraceptives that employ the oral route of administration have the disadvantage that the drug has to go through the gastrointestinal (GI) tract, which can result in diminished efficacy due to diarrhoea or vomiting. In addition, the daily intake of tablets results in daily peak concentrations.

Non-oral routes of administration offer the possibility of being able to use lower doses of hormones while still achieving adequate contraceptive efficacy and good cycle control. The contraceptive controlled-release formulations that are currently on the market are progestogen-only products such as injectables, the IUS and implants. However, all these methods are associated with disrupted cycle control. Another disadvantage is that they involve an injection or a minor surgical procedure.

Both EVRA and the NuvaRing are combined oestrogen-progestogen contraceptives, which guarantee ovulation inhibition and share the following advantages:

- continuous release of hormones, thereby avoiding high peak concentrations;
- avoidance of absorption via the gastrointestinal tract and the hepatic first-pass effect, which allows lower dosing, and removes the necessity for extra precautions during GI upsets. In addition, (although recommended by some) it should no longer be necessary to advise

extra precautions during the use of broad-spectrum antibiotics (but these will continue to be necessary with enzyme-inducing drugs) (Abrams *et al.* 2002; Dogterom *et al.* 2005);

- no need to remember daily administration;
- the woman has full control over her contraceptive method.

The EVRA patch

EVRA, a contraceptive patch containing 20 μg of ethinylestradiol and 150 μg of norelgestromin (the primary active metabolite of norgestimate), was launched in the UK in 2003. Each patch is worn for a week for three consecutive weeks followed by one patch-free week. The patch can be placed on the buttocks, abdomen, the back or the upper arm (but not on the breasts). Showering, bathing and swimming do not appear to affect adherence. A study has even looked at women wearing their patch in a sauna and exercising in a gym, and these activities did not significantly affect adherence (Zacur *et al.* 2002). In the clinical trials, approximately 17% of women experienced mild to moderate application site reactions, but only 2% discontinued the method for this reason (Sibai *et al.* 2002).

Studies in Europe and North America have shown high efficacy, with the method failure being between 0.4 and 0.99 per 100 woman-years and the user failure between 0.7 and 1.24 per 100 woman-years (Audet *et al.* 2001; Smallwood *et al.* 2001). There is a suggestion that efficacy may be reduced in women who weigh more than 90 kg, since a third of failures (5 out of 15) have occurred in such women (who only constituted 3% of the study population). The reasons for this are not entirely clear; it is noteworthy that four out of the five women weighing more than 90 kg who became pregnant were from the USA and participated in the same study (Smallwood *et al.* 2001). However, this should not be an important issue, since most women who weigh more than 90 kg will have a BMI greater than 30 [unless they are over 5 ft 10 inches (1.78 m) tall], and thus should not be using an oestrogen-containing contraceptive (see Chapter 9).

Cycle control was good and comparable to that of Trinordiol and Mercilon (Audet *et al.* 2001), though more women using the patch had spotting in the first two cycles (approximately 10% of women had spotting or bleeding in the third cycle). The main side effect was transient breast tenderness in the first couple of months, experienced by

22% of users, but only 2% discontinued the studies for this reason. Women put on an average of 0.4 kg over a year, regardless of whether they were using the patch or Trinordiol.

Compliance with the patch regimen has been shown to be better than with an oral contraceptive, particularly in young women. Only 68% of women under the age of 20 took their pills correctly, compared with 88% of those using a patch (Archer *et al.* 2002). Since compliance affects efficacy, the patch is likely to be a useful alternative for those who find it difficult to remember a daily pill.

NuvaRing

NuvaRing is a vaginal ring containing 15 μg of ethinylestradiol and 120 μg of etonorgestrel (3-ketodesogestrel). It has been available for some time in many European countries, including Eire, although it is not yet available in the UK. It is hoped that it will be launched in the UK in the next couple of years. The ring is flexible and transparent; it is made of ethylene vinylacetate (EVA) copolymers, with an outer diameter of 54 mm and a cross-sectional diameter of 4 mm.

Each ring is to be used for 3 weeks, followed by a one-week ring-free interval. Like the EVRA patch, NuvaRing can be inserted and removed by the woman herself. In a large multicentre trial (Dieben *et al.* 2002) the method failure was 0.77 per 100 woman-years, and the user failure rate was 1.18 per 100 woman-years.

NuvaRing has particularly good cycle control. Breakthrough bleeding (which is mostly spotting) occurs in less than 6% of cycles, even in the initial months of use (Dieben *et al.* 2002). Comparative trials suggest that the bleeding pattern in women using NuvaRing is even better than with Microgynon (probably because blood levels of hormone are less variable).

NuvaRing appears to have a safety margin for delayed replacement of up to 7 days, in terms of efficacy, but a study investigating this aspect found that cycle control was reduced. Thus, if a woman wishes to avoid her withdrawal bleeds, she should put a new ring in after 3 weeks, and not increase the duration of use of the old one. Vaginally administered antimycotics and spermicides are unlikely to affect the contraceptive efficacy and safety of NuvaRing.

The ring can be removed for intercourse if desired, but must be reinserted within 3 hours afterwards. If the ring has been outside the vagina for more than 3 hours, contraceptive efficacy may be reduced.

The ring should be reinserted as soon as possible and barrier method should be used in addition until the NuvaRing has been used continuously for 7 days.

There is a rapid return of fertility following removal of the NuvaRing (within the first month). No significant changes have been observed in blood pressure, weight, or metabolic parameters in women using NuvaRing. The most commonly reported side effect related to the ring was non-specific vaginitis, which occurred in 6% of women, though only 1% withdrew from the studies for this reason.

The acceptability of NuvaRing use was investigated in the large multicentre studies in the USA, Canada and Europe (Novak *et al.* 2003). The main reasons most frequently mentioned for liking NuvaRing were 'not having to remember anything' (43%), 'easy to use' (28%) and 'an effective method' (10%). The main reason given for not liking NuvaRing was 'interference with intercourse'. Almost all the women were very satisfied with the use of the ring, preferred it to other methods of contraception and would recommend it to others.

Further into the future

Combined oestrogen-progestogen injectables

Lunelle (previously called Cyclofem), a combination of medroxyprogesterone acetate (25 mg) and oestradiol cypionate (5 mg) in a 0.5 ml dose, is a new injectable contraceptive that has been successfully used in worldwide trials and may be marketed in the UK in the next couple of years. WHO studies have shown first-year failure rates of 0.2 per 100 woman-years (Upadhyay 2005). An advantage of this preparation is that there is far less menstrual disturbance than with progestogen-only injectables (Upadhyay 2005). However, the injections have to be given monthly, which is clearly inconvenient for many women. Self-injection appears to be a viable option, and has recently been approved by the United States FDA (Upadhyay 2005).

Male hormonal contraception

The 'male pill' may not be a figment of our imagination for much longer. Various combinations of androgen-only and androgen-progestogen combinations are under investigation. However, an actual pill has been difficult to produce and it is likely that the first versions will be injections or subcutaneous pellets. Although there has been much scepticism about the acceptability of a male pill, there is also a more general feeling that contraceptive responsibility should be shared and many men in stable relationships appear to be keen to take part.

References and further reading

Abrams LS, Skee D, Natarajan J, Wong FA. (2002) Pharmacokinetic overview of Ortho Evra(tm)/Evra. *Fertil Steril* **77**(Suppl 2), S3–12.

Archer DF, Bigrigg A, Smallwood GH, Shangol GA, Creasy GW, Fisher AC. (2002) Assessment of compliance with a weekly contraceptive patch (Ortho EVRA/EVRA) among North American women. *Fertil Steril* **77**(2), Suppl 2, S27–31.

Audet M, Moreau M, Koltun WD *et al.* (2001) Evaluation of contraceptive efficacy and cycle control of a transdermal contraceptive patch vs an oral contraceptive: a randomized control trial. *J Am Med Assoc* **285**, 2347–54.

Dieben TOM, Roumen FJM, Apter D. (2002) Efficacy, cycle control and user acceptability of a novel combined contraceptive vaginal ring. *Hum Reprod* **100**(3), 585–93.

Dogterom P, van den Heuvel MW, Thomsen T. (2005) Absence of pharmacokinetic interactions of the combined contraceptive vaginal ring NuvaRing with oral amoxicillin or doxycycline in two randomised trials. *Clin Pharmacokinet* **44**(4), 429–38.

Foidart J-M, Wuttke W, Bouw GM, Gertlinger C, Heithecker R. (2000) A comparative investigation of contraceptive reliability, cycle control and tolerance of two monophasic oral contraceptives containing either drospirenone or desogestrel. *Eur J Contracept Reprod Health Care* **5**(2), 124–34.

Glasier A. (1997) Emergency postcoital contraception. *N Engl J Med* **337**, 1058–64.

Heinemann LAJ, Dinger J. (2004) Safety of a new oral contraceptive containing drospirenone. *Drug Safety* **27** (13), 1001–18.

Huber J, Foidart J-M, Wuttke W *et al.* (2000) Efficacy and tolerability of a monophasic oral contraceptive containing ethinyloestradiol and drospirenone. *Eur J Contracept Reprod Health Care* **5**(1), 25–34.

Korver T, Dieben T, Vree M, Van Muijen AE, Vromans L, Van Der Sanden A, Van Osta G. (1998) A double blind study comparing the contraceptive efficacy, acceptability and safety of two progestogen-only pills containing desogestrel 75 mcg/day or levonorgestrel 30 mcg/day. *Eur J Contracept Reprod Health Care* **3**, 169–78.

Korver T, Klipping C, Heger-Mahn D, Duijkers I, van Osta G, Dieben T. (2005) Maintenance of ovulation inhibition with the 75-microg desogestrel-only contraceptive pill (Cerazette) after scheduled 12-h delays in tablet intake. *Contraception* **71**(1), 8–13.

Novak A, de la Logeb C, Abetzc L, van der Meulena EA. (2003) The combined contraceptive vaginal ring, NuvaRing: an international study of user acceptability. *Contraception* **67**, 187–94.
Oelkers W, Foidart J-M, Dombrovicz N *et al.* (1995) Effects of a new oral contraceptive containing an antimineralocorticoid progestogen, drospirenone, on the renin-aldosterone system, body weight, blood pressure, glucose tolerance and lipid metabolism. *J Clin Endocrinol Metab* **80**(6), 1816–21.
Parsey KS, Pong A. (2000) An open-label, multicentre study to evaluate Yasmin, a low dose combination oral contraceptive containing drospirenone, a new progestogen. *Contraception* **61**(2), 105–11.
Rice C, Killick SR, Dieben T, Coehlingh Bennink H. (1999) A comparison of the inhibition of ovulation achieved by desogestrel 75 mcg and levonorgestrel 30 mcg daily. *Hum Reprod* **14**(4), 982–5.
Roumen FJME, Apter D, Mulders TMT, Dieben TOM. (2001) Efficacy, tolerability and acceptability of a novel contraceptive vaginal ring releasing etonorgestrel and ethinyl oestradiol. *Hum Reprod* **16**, 469–75.
Sibai BM, Odlind V, Meador ML, Shangold GA, Fisher AC, Creasy GW. (2002) A comparative and pooled analysis of the safety and tolerability of the contraceptive patch (Ortho EVRA/EVRA). *Fertil Steril* **77**(2), Suppl 2, S19–26.
Smallwood GH, Meador M, Lenihan JP, Shangold GA, Fisher AC, Creasy GW. (2001) Efficacy and safety of a transdermal contraceptive system. *Obstet Gynecol* **98**, 799–805.
Upadhyay, UD. (2005) *New contraceptive choices.* Population Reports, Series M, No. 19. The INFO Project. Baltimore: Johns Hopkins Bloomberg School of Public Health.
Van Vloten WA, van Haselen CW, van Zuuren EJ, Gerlinger C, Heithecker R. (2002) The effect of two combined oral contraceptives containing either drospirenone or cyproterone acetate on acne and seborrhea. *Cutis* **69**(4S), 2–15.
Vessey M. (2001) Oral contraceptive failures and body weight: findings in a large cohort study. *J Fam Plann Reprod Health Care* **27**(2), 90–1.
Von Hertzen H, Piaggio G, Ding J, *et al.* for the WHO research group on postovulatory methods of fertility regulation (2002). Low dose mifepristone and two regimens of levonorgestrel for emergency contraception: a WHO multicentre randomized trial. *Lancet* **360**, 1803–10.
WHO Task Force on Postovulatory Methods of Fertility Regulation. (1999) Comparison of three single doses of mifepristone as emergency contraception: a randomised trial. *Lancet* **353**, 697–702.
Webb AMC. (2003) Emergency contraception. *Br Med J* **326**, 775-6.
Zacur HA, Hedon B, Mansour D, Shangold GA, Fisher AC, Creasy GW. (2002) Integrated summary of Ortho EVRA/EVRA contraceptive patch adhesion in varied climates and conditions. *Fertil Steril* **77**(2), Suppl 2, S32–5.

PART 2

CONTRACEPTION IN DIFFERENT USER GROUPS

7 CONTRACEPTION FOR YOUNG PEOPLE

Sexuality and young people

Debate about teenage sexuality was noted as early as the seventeenth century by Shakespeare in Romeo and Juliet:

CAPULET: My child is yet a stranger in the world,
She hath not seen the change of fourteen years;
Let two more summers wither in their pride
Ere we may think her ripe to be a bride.
PARIS: Younger than she are happy mothers made.
CAPULET: And too soon marr'd are those so early made.

However, in Shakespeare's day, human physiology itself resulted in the problem being a smaller one than it is now. It has been calculated that in 1870 only approximately 13% of girls were fully fertile by the age of 17.5 years, while in 1970 the figure was approximately 94%. Improved nutritional standards are thought to have been responsible for the gradual decline in the age of menarche over the last two centuries: in Britain in the year 1900 the average age of menarche was 14.0 years, while by 1960, it had come down to 12.9 years. An earlier menarche, and therefore earlier development of secondary sexual characteristics, leads not only to an earlier awareness of sexuality, but also enables pregnancy to occur at a younger age. The fact is that today's teenagers are becoming physically sexually mature at a younger age than ever before. This fact cannot be ignored, especially since the result has been a widening discrepancy between the adolescent's knowledge about sexual matters and the physical possibilities. The subject of teenage sexuality has been much in the news during the last few years. A great deal has been said regarding its acceptability or otherwise. Table 7.1 shows the percentage of males and females with experience of sexual intercourse at different ages.

Corresponding with the falling age at menarche, there has been an increase in teenage sexual activity. While the incidence of sexual activity has risen for both sexes and all ages, the greatest increase has been in the group of 16-year-old girls.

Table 7.1 Percentage of males and females with experience of SI at different ages

Age	Males (%)			Females (%)		
	1964	1974	1989	1964	1974	1989
16	14	32	53	5	21	51
17	26	50	67	10	37	67
18	34	65	83	17	47	83

Combination of Bury J (1984) More teenage sex. *Teenage pregnancy in Britain.* London: Birth Control Trust, page 33; and Ford N. (1992) The sexual and contraceptive lifestyles of young people: part 1. *Br J Fam Plann* **18**, 52–5.

Thus more teenagers are having sexual intercourse, and at a younger age than in the past. However, this does not necessarily imply that they have become more promiscuous. As is always the case, the public image of the extreme minority tends to mask the moderate majority. The predominant form of sexual behaviour amongst teenage girls during the last 30 years has been that of 'serial monogamy', i.e. one faithful, stable relationship becomes replaced, after a period of time, with

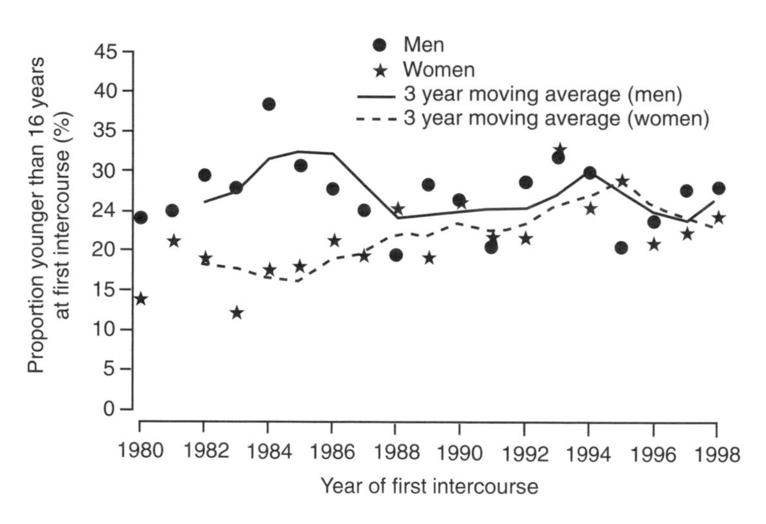

Figure 7.1 Proportion of participants younger than 16 years at first intercourse, by year of first intercourse. Modified from Wellings K *et al.* (2001) Sexual behaviour in Britain: early heterosexual experience. *Lancet* **358**, 1843–50.

another. At this point, it is necessary to distinguish between older teenagers and younger teenagers. Older teenagers, over the age of 17, in general are comparable to women in their early 20s. It is the younger group, and of course, in particular, the under 16s, who are usually referred to when 'teenage sexuality' is discussed. This is not without foundation, as it is the 'younger adolescent' who is least prepared, both emotionally and intellectually, for a sexual relationship and its implications. A number of studies have pointed out that the ability to think in conceptual, non-egocentric, future-oriented terms is not possible until the middle or late stages of adolescence. With increasing age there develops the ability to grasp the concept that a sexual relationship involves another person with feelings, values and expectations of his or her own, that pregnancy could result and that contraception is necessary to prevent pregnancy (Blos, 1972; Chilman 1979).

This age-related development disadvantages many young people and should be borne in mind when assessing their needs. How can we account for the increase in teenage sexual activity? Earlier sexual maturation is not enough to explain the dramatic rise in the last 30 years. The answers lie in the social environment in which teenagers have been, and are being brought up. Ever since the end of the Second World War there has been a trend towards relaxation of attitudes towards both social and sexual behaviour; this reached its peak during the 'swinging sixties and seventies'. Children and teenagers growing up during this time were naturally influenced by the more liberal adult attitudes and behaviour. At the same time, rising divorce rates (now one in three marriages) resulted in diminished parental discipline, a factor that has been shown to be associated with adolescent sexual experience. The influence of the media, coupled with the decline in the influence of religion, cannot be ignored. By 1972, an American study concluded that television had replaced the church as society's strongest influence on young people (Rubenstein *et al.* 1972). The advertising industry has exploited teenagers' worries about their appearance, promoting acne remedies and beauty aids. Sexual relationships/attractiveness are often an underlying theme in these adverts. Teenagers are increasingly exposed to 'glamorous sex' both on television and in films. They can read the latest real-life scandals in the newspapers every day. Wherever they look, they are given the impression that 'everyone is doing it' and, what is more, that everyone is doing it without contraception. The actual extent of the influence that the media exerts is the subject of debate, but its importance cannot be denied. It is sad that we have had to wait for a fatal sexually transmitted disease to make people wake up to the possibility of using the media in a positive way. Now, at long last, the word 'condom' is permissible on TV, at long last they are allowed to be advertised. In addition to the 'sex is okay' message, today's society is also giving another very negative message that implies that behaviour that is okay when you are 40 is not okay when you are only 16. This mixed message is often resented by young people and leads to a lack of trust of authority.

Sexual ill health in teenagers

Sexually transmitted infections

The prevalence of sexually transmitted infections (STIs) amongst young people in the UK is increasing. In all age groups there was an increase in gonorrhoea by 58% and chlamydia by 76% in the second half of the 1990s. The biggest increase was in those under 25.

Unplanned pregnancy

Given that there has been an increase in teenage sexual activity, it is not surprising that teenage pregnancy rates have also risen (Figure 7.2).

Teenage pregnancy rates reached a peak in the early 1970s and the trend until 1984 was generally downward. The pregnancy rate per 1000 women aged 15–19 was 63 in 1971 compared to 49 in 1985, a fall of 14. One would expect an increase in sexual activity to be associated with an increase in the pregnancy rate, but on the contrary, the pregnancy rate decreased. The rise in the abortion rate was not enough to account for the drop in the live-birth rate. The fact is that teenagers were using contraception. The fall in the pregnancy rate coincided with the free availability of contraception to all women, in 1974. It can be seen that the pregnancy rate began to fall in the mid-1970s, at the time contraception became more easily available. In addition, there was a gradual shift of emphasis from the condom and withdrawal (both non-medical methods) to the combined oral contraceptive pill (available on prescription only). A great deal of harm was wrought by the case of Mrs Victoria Gillick vs West Norfolk and Wisbech AHA and DHSS. In December 1984, a Court of Appeal decided in favour of Mrs Gillick,

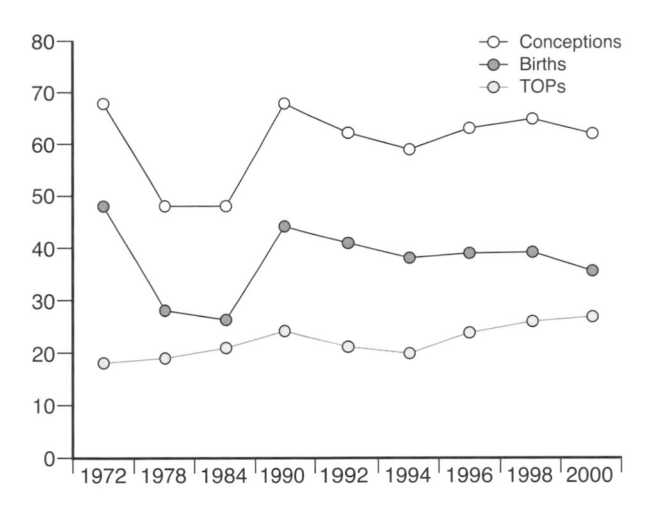

Figure 7.2 Birth, termination of pregnancy (TOP) and conception rates in 15–19-year-olds, 1972–2000 (/1000). Source: Office of National Statistics, 2000.

who had insisted that none of her daughters under the age of 16 should be given contraceptive advice without her prior knowledge and consent. The DHSS immediately appealed to the House of Lords, but it was 9 months before the case was judged and essentially overthrown.

Box 7.1 Fraser Guidelines 1985 for treating under-16s. All conditions must apply for consent to be given

- The doctor must try to persuade her to inform her parents.
- The client must have sufficient maturity to understand the advice.
- The client must be likely to begin or continue sexual intercourse without contraception.
- Without contraception, the client's physical or mental health may suffer.
- It is in the client's best interests to give contraceptive advice and/or treatment without parental consent.

Adapted from 'Confidentiality and people under 16'. Guidance issued jointly by the BMA, GMS, HEA, Brook, FPA and RCGP.

During that 9 months, the Court of Appeal's judgment was law. This meant that it was illegal to prescribe contraception to under-age girls 'save in emergency'. This clause was variously interpreted by individual doctors. However, it was widely assumed by teenagers that if they asked for contraception, they would be turned down and worse, their parents would automatically be informed. Not surprisingly, attendance by under-16s at the Brook Advisory Clinics dropped by nearly 40%. Eventually a ruling was issued which essentially stated that people under 16 years of age are legally able to consent on their own behalf to any surgical or medical procedure or treatment if, in the doctor's opinion, they are capable of understanding the nature and possible consequences of the procedure. It is recommended that good clinical notes be kept. There are several issues a doctor should consider and these are shown in Box 7.1.

Improving sexual ill health in young people

Unfortunately, the most important factors are all social ones. A number of authors have pointed out that for a young girl from a poor socio-economic background with few prospects, pregnancy may be viewed as the most rewarding of the options available. This will naturally influence, consciously or subconsciously, her motivation to use birth control. It follows that if teenage pregnancy rates are to be reduced, the alternatives must be made more attractive. Improved sex education and education in general are clearly important. Studies in the USA have shown that improving teenagers' social prospects through education and career goals and opportunities is a very important factor in the prevention of both initial and repeat pregnancies.

Providing sex education in schools, along with general health education, is important. A very successful scheme used the school health service to provide contraceptive advice, smears and so on. The big advantage is that the school nurse does not change frequently, and knows the pupils for a long time.

In a school in Minnesota, such a scheme led to a halving of the pregnancy rate within 3 years. The country that has had the best results in reducing teenage pregnancy is the Netherlands (see Figure 7.3). What they have done is actually quite simple. Over a 20-year period, the government has provided sex education from an early age (starting in primary schools at age 6), combined with easily accessible contracep-

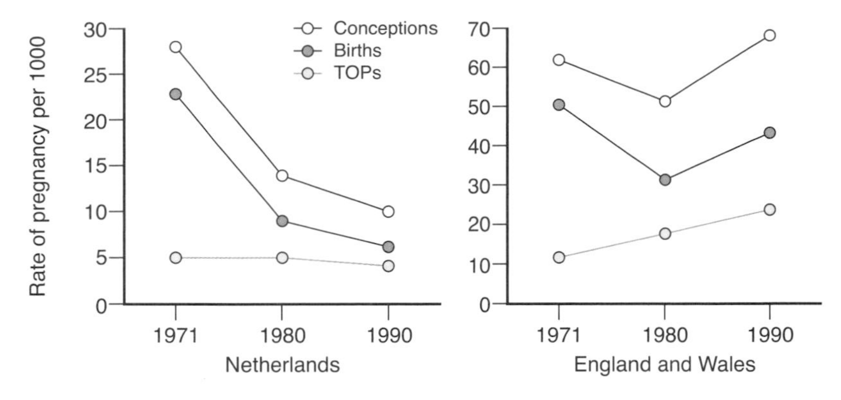

Figure 7.3 Pregnancy rates per 1000 15–19-year-olds. TOP, termination of pregnancy.

tive and abortion services. In addition, there is an openness about sexuality in the Netherlands which means that teenagers are not exposed to conflicting messages. The media have also had an important part to play in this, as they have been much more honest and responsible in the depiction of sex and contraceptive issues (Box 7.2).

In the UK, many people throw their hands up in horror at the thought of sex education and contraceptive advice for teenagers. There is a point of view that states that if young people are 'forbidden' to have sexual intercourse, given very limited sex education, and refused contraception, they will be discouraged from intercourse, and pregnancy and sexually transmitted disease rates will fall accordingly. In fact, there is

Box 7.2 The Dutch model

- Liberal family attitudes to contraception and sexuality
- Responsible media programmes and articles
- Outreach workers visit schools, youth clubs, Church groups and parents' organizations
- Free, confidential, easily accessible clinics

From Williams E. (1994) Contraceptive compliance among young people. *Br J Sex Med* **May/June**.

no evidence that knowledge leads to earlier or increased sexual activity. On the contrary, in the Netherlands, the age at first intercourse has actually risen, as has the number of teenagers using contraception at first intercourse.

A report published by the Alan Guttmacher Institute in 1985 compared the factors associated with teenage pregnancy in six Western countries in 1980. The pregnancy rate was highest in the USA, at 96 per 1000 15–19-year-olds and lowest in Holland, at 14 per 1000 15–19-year-olds. In England and Wales the rate was 44 (Jones *et al.* 1985). In 1986, Francome published a comparison of abortion practices in 1984 in Britain and the USA. The abortion rate in the USA was twice that in England and Wales. Both Francome's study and the Guttmacher report have highlighted lack of sex education and the influence of conflicting messages about sex as being important contributory factors to the high pregnancy rates, and therefore abortion rates, in the USA.

In Holland, sex education concerns itself mainly with biological facts, but contraceptive education is managed by government-subsidized specialized mobile teams. In addition, they have greatly increased the use of the media in responsibly promoting contraception and knowledge of sexual matters. In the USA, the combination of varying degrees of religious views and different laws in different states has led to a patchy, and, in general, poorly co-ordinated service, both in terms of education and provision of contraception. In addition, the effect of the media in 'glamorizing' sex, as mentioned earlier, appears to be particularly strong in the USA.

There are conflicting views as to who should be responsible for sex education: should it be the school or the parents? It would seem in everyone's best interests if the responsibility were shared. So far, studies have suggested that, with some excellent exceptions, neither parents nor schools appear to be imparting much useful knowledge to teenagers, who rely, as always, mainly on information from friends and peers. This is worrying, as such information is likely to be the least reliable.

At present in the UK, although by law some form of sex education has to be provided by schools, all details are left to the discretion of the governing bodies; parents must be informed of the content of the lessons. Often teachers have had little training to give sex education, and the quality and content appear to vary enormously from school to school. The unfortunate result is that in some schools sex education is scanty or poorly presented. There is surely a need for carefully considered national guidelines as to form and content, which should take into account differing cultural and religious views.

A number of surveys have shown that an overwhelming majority of parents are in favour of sex education in principle, and indeed, often feel there is not enough. In addition, a number of studies have shown that teenagers do not receive sex education early enough: both Francome (1986) and Simms and Smith (1986) have shown that a significant number of teenagers are actually already sexually active by the time they receive any instruction about relationships or birth control. The USA, which has the greatest problems in this area, has been carrying out a considerable amount of research to try and find solutions. Varying types of structured sex education programmes have (and are) being tried. In general, it has been found that young people respond better to discussions in small groups, and appear to be influenced particularly when role-playing techniques are used. It is stressed that the most successful teaching is done in 'programmes' extending over several weeks or more. In addition, it seems important that at least some of the discussions should take place in mixed groups, to encourage an outlook of shared responsibility. Participation with involvement of parents is beneficial.

Access to services and contraceptive use

In order to understand teenagers' use of and preferences in contraception, it is necessary to look at the nature of their sexual activity and their attitudes towards it. For the majority of teenagers, sexual intercourse is infrequent and unplanned, especially at the beginning of a relationship. Numerous studies have shown that more than 50% of teenage first sexual encounters occur without the use of contraception. It is also well established that the less stable a relationship is, the less likely it is that contraception will be used. This curious logic is not exclusive to teenagers. Part of the problem for young girls appears to lie in the conflict between having sex but avoiding appearing 'cheap'. Premarital sex is still subject to the age-old double standard, whereby the young man is merely 'sowing wild oats' while a young woman doing the same is considered promiscuous. Some young women therefore feel that if they are unprepared for sex they will be viewed more kindly than if they have obviously planned ahead by using contraception.

Teenagers are often poorly informed and are susceptible to 'myths' such as 'pregnancy will not occur if intercourse is infrequent' or 'a girl can only become pregnant if she has an orgasm' and so on. It has been shown in countries such as Holland that, where sex education is the norm, teenagers have a more informed attitude towards sex and contraception. The attitude of young men towards contraception is often just as confused as that of young women. They too feel that contraception is less important in a casual relationship. The advent of the pill has tended to shift responsibility physically on to the female partner and with it has gone the need for responsible behaviour/attitude by the man. In addition, young men often lack the confidence to both buy and use sheaths.

A further problem which besets contraceptive use, not least by teenagers, is poor motivation. Most contraceptive methods require continuing motivation, to use a barrier method consistently, or to take a pill regularly. This requires a degree of responsibility and self-control which teenagers often lack. They are also more likely to be influenced by 'scares' and side effects, and have a tendency to discontinue their method without first considering alternatives. The teenager's attitude and perception of pregnancy and motherhood may also influence motivation. A teenage girl with few social/career prospects may perceive motherhood as being a way of achieving some kind of status and fulfilment.

Access to contraception and advice can be difficult for teenagers and is often not made easy by the healthcare system itself. They may feel embarrassed to talk to their GP who has known them as children, and who also knows their parents. They may worry about being seen by their parents' friends, their own friends, or neighbours in a clinic. In the last few years there has been a great deal of publicity relating to the confidentiality and legality of contraceptive and sexual health consultations for the under-16s. This may deter an anxious teenager who does not fully understand the current position. Counselling teenagers is not easy and requires a sympathetic attitude and, occasionally, patience. If a young woman suffers either psychologically or physically in the initial stages of her contraceptive experience, she is much less likely to be motivated and to access services in the future.

When a teenager comes for contraceptive advice, she may wish to ask more general questions about sex and relationships, and these should be dealt with in a sympathetic, non-judgemental manner. This is, however, an opportunity to discuss the problems of adolescent sex with her, and the younger she is, the more important this aspect becomes. Early age at first intercourse has long been associated with an increased risk of cervical cancer, and this is only one of the many sexually transmitted diseases of which the teenager may be at risk, whether bacterial (chlamydia, gonococcus) or viral [hepatitis B, human immunodeficiency virus (HIV)]. It is difficult to try and explain such future-oriented problems to teenagers, especially younger teenagers, and especially difficult to do so without sounding pompous and judgemental. The launch of the Chlamydia Awareness Campaign in the UK in 2002 may have made this easier. It is also essential not to miss the small number of teenage girls who have come ostensibly to discuss contraception, perhaps being subject to peer-group pressure, but in reality are seeking 'permission' to refrain from intercourse at that time.

Methods

When considering methods of contraception for teenagers, it is more important than usual to bear in mind that the best method for any individual is the one she finds most acceptable, involving her partner also whenever appropriate. The ideal contraceptive (see Box 7.3) does not exist, nor is it likely to exist in the near future. Therefore, the advantages and disadvantages of any particular method must be assessed for each individual and the eventual choice will be the 'least bad'.

Box 7.3 Characteristics of the ideal contraceptive method for teenagers

- No side effects
- Independent of user's motivation/skill in use
- Independent of intercourse
- Very effective protection against pregnancy
- Suitable for infrequent, unplanned intercourse
- Protective against all varieties of sexually transmitted disease
- No health risks
- Cheap and easily available, without need for medical supervision
- Easily and completely reversible

The use of contraception varies with age and the duration of the relationship (Figures 7.4 and 7.5). Young people rely more on barriers than older teenagers who are more likely to use a more effective method. This may be related to access to methods. Earlier in a relationship condoms are the method most likely to be used and oral contraceptives in longer duration relationships. However, 30% use no contraception at all.

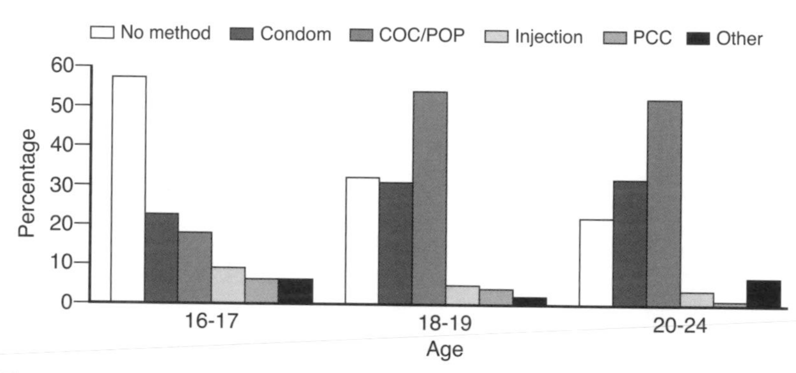

Figure 7.4 Contraceptive methods used by teenagers/young people (%). Source: Office of National Statistics, 2000 (Great Britain). COC, combined oral contraceptive; POP, progestogen-only pill; PCC, post-coital contraception.

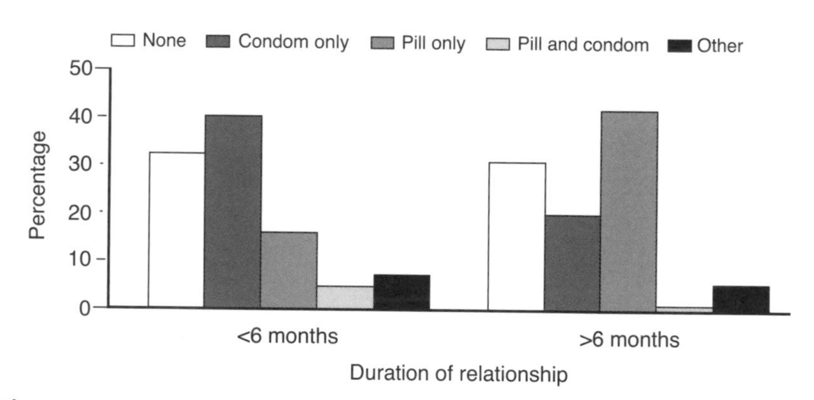

Figure 7.5 Contraceptive method used and last intercourse by duration of current sexual relationship (%). Source: Wellings K. (1986) Trends in contraceptive method usage since 1970. *Br J Fam Plann* **12**, 57–64.

The combined oral contraceptive (COC) pill and the EVRA patch

Despite all the pill scares, this remains the most popular method of contraception amongst teenagers. The pill hardly seems an ideal method for women who are having infrequent intercourse. However, it has other important advantages, namely that it is very effective, is not intercourse related and is reasonably easy to use. It has a protective effect against pelvic inflammatory disease (PID), which is an advantage for teenagers. The pill also solves the problem of irregular, heavy, painful periods, from which many teenagers suffer. Indeed, teenagers often use this as a covert request for contraception. There is no evidence that the pill inhibits growth in teenagers, as was once suggested. Studies in young animals showed that high doses of oestrogen could cause premature closure of the epiphyses. However, there is no evidence that the amounts used even in higher-dose combined pills have this effect. By the time menstruation is established, growth is already more or less complete.

Unfortunately, teenagers are the group most adversely affected by the October 1995 pill scare regarding the risk of venous thrombosis (Figure 7.6). They are the largest group of first-time users, and the first-time user

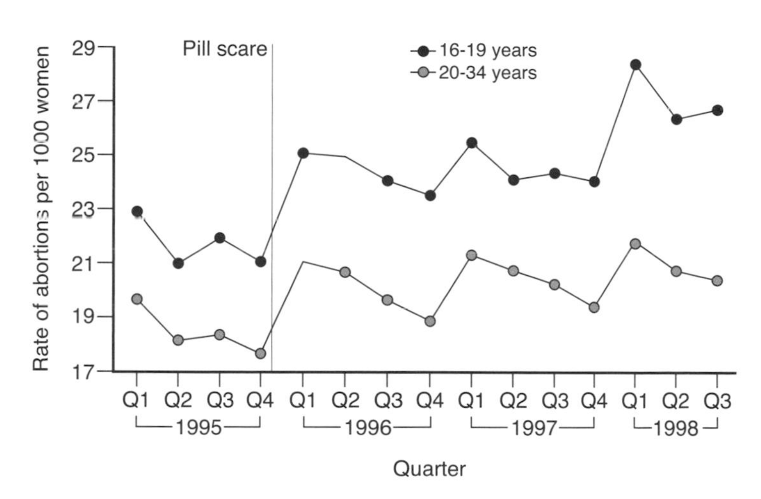

Figure 7.6 The abortion rate before and after the 'Pill scare': 16–34-year-olds. Source: Office of National Statistics.

is the one most likely to have deep vein thrombosis (DVT), regardless of which pill she is on. However, because of the Committee on the Safety of Medicine (CSM) ruling, in 1995, the Faculty of Family Planning and Reproductive Health Care suggested that first-time users should preferentially be given second-generation pills, unless there was a reason, including acne, for choosing a third-generation pill.

That mention of acne is important in this context. Many teenagers are obsessed with their appearance and may benefit from a third-generation pill. If so, the Faculty guidelines have always allowed you to prescribe them. Another is Cilest, which was not mentioned in the CSM letter. And in fact, a triphasic version of Cilest was given a licence for the treatment of acne by the Food and Drug Administration (FDA) in January 1997. The issue of the COC and venous thromboembolism (VTE) is dealt with in Chapter 9 and will not be discussed further here.

Taking the pill requires a regular routine and continuing motivation, which are both drawbacks for teenagers. There is a tendency to discontinue the method abruptly when a relationship ends, or runs into problems. In addition, side effects or bad publicity regarding the pill may result in a teenager stopping it before obtaining an alternative method. For this reason, it is helpful to explain the possible side effects when a teenager first starts the pill, and to point out that there are many different formulations to try if the first one does not suit. Everyday (ED) packs may be useful for the teenager who finds the pill-taking regimen difficult to manage. The EVRA patch has been shown to have significantly better compliance than the pill in teenagers, which may make it a useful alternative. It has all the advantages of the pill for teenagers, but without the need to remember a pill every day.

Condoms

Although this method is still the most commonly used at the start of a relationship, it has tended to be rapidly replaced by the pill. In theory, the sheath perhaps comes closest to fulfilling the requirements of the 'ideal' contraceptive for teenagers. It is well suited to infrequent intercourse. It protects against many sexually transmitted infections. It has no side effects or health risks, does not affect fertility and does not require medical supervision.

Unfortunately, the effective use of condoms requires a confidence and expertise that young men often lack. In addition, obtaining them is fraught with difficulties for the young, embarrassed teenager. Young men are understandably reluctant to enter the female-dominated family planning clinics and so the increasing tendency for GPs to provide free condoms is important. Buying sheaths at the chemist can also be embarrassing, especially if the assistant is female. Sheaths can be obtained from barbers and vending machines, which appear to be more acceptable sources, although we have yet to see the latter in schools.

Condoms have become more respectable as a result of the AIDS (acquired immunodeficiency syndrome) publicity, but unfortunately, the message that appears to have got through is 'use a condom instead of the pill' as opposed to 'as well as'. Young people in particular are likely to experience a high failure rate using condoms, through a combination of high fertility and lack of experience in their use. We should be trying to promote the 'double Dutch' method of both pill and condom together.

The diaphragm, like the sheath, is suitable for infrequent intercourse. However, teenagers often find the idea distasteful and the practice messy and inconvenient. Given the often rather unplanned, secretive and hasty nature of teenage sexual intercourse, a method that involves premeditation, a meticulous insertion technique, a need for washing facilities and a bulky container is hardly likely to achieve popularity. It is not surprising that studies have shown high failure rates in young people. Spermicides also tend to be regarded as messy and unreliable.

Intrauterine methods of contraception

The NICE guideline does not identify any contraindications to intrauterine device (IUD) use in young or in nulliparous women specifically, indeed it has several advantages for young people, namely that it is very effective, is not intercourse related and does not require continuing motivation. On the other side of the argument there are disadvantages, which individual women need to consider before using the method.

The infection rate and expulsion rates of IUDs are highest in young women. The increased infection rate is a reflection of the prevalence of STI at this young age. The incidence of PID in IUD users is approximately double that of users of no contraception and is only increased for the first 20 days after insertion, thereafter the rate equals the background rate. However, in the absence of an STI, an IUD is not contraindicated on grounds of age or parity alone as the risk of PID is extremely low.

For some young women the Mirena intrauterine system (IUS) is a better choice than the copper IUD. It is even more effective than a copper IUD and makes periods lighter and less painful. However, bleeding is still likely to be irregular, which may not be well tolerated. In addition, the use of local anaesthetic for the fitting may sometimes be required in nulliparous women.

Injectable contraceptives

Injectable progestogens have several advantages for young women: they are highly effective, independent of user motivation and of intercourse and offer protection against PID. In many ways they offer the advantages of the IUD without the risk of infection, or the trauma of insertion. Unfortunately, they also have several disadvantages, which put teenagers off. Teenagers are not likely to tolerate very irregular bleeding. Also, the possibility of weight gain is unpopular when teenagers are already so anxious about appearance. However, increasingly, it is seen by many young people as an acceptable and effective method of contraception. Good counselling and support if bleeding problems occur are important to ensure continued use of this very effective method. Attainment of peak bone mass has emerged as a concern in the last few years: this is discussed in Chapter 3.

Subdermal implants

Implanon is an implant which consists of a single, semi-rigid rod, measuring 40 mm by 2 mm. It releases 30–40 µg of etonorgestrel (3 ketodesogestrel) per day and lasts for 3 years. This hormone level is designed to achieve complete inhibition of ovulation and so far, in the worldwide phase III clinical trials, there has not been a single pregnancy.

The implant comes preloaded in a disposable inserter, which is about the same size as a blood transfusion needle, and the insertion procedure is very simple, not requiring a skin incision. Insertion takes, on average, 2 minutes. Removal, using a 'pop-out' technique, is facilitated by the rigidity of the capsule and takes 3 minutes. Implanon is rapidly reversible: within a week of removal, blood levels of hormone are undetectable.

Amenorrhoea is more common in Implanon users than with Norplant (21% versus 10%, respectively). However, there is no evidence that hypo-oestrogenicity is a problem in Implanon users. Etonorgestrel appears to inhibit luteinizing hormone (LH), but not follicle-stimulating hormone (FSH), so follicles, and therefore oestradiol, are still produced. The incidence of acne appears to be slightly lower than with the levonorgestrel implants. However, irregular bleeding can be a problem, as with all progestogen-only methods.

Progestogen-only pill (POP)

The POP in general is not very suitable for teenagers. It relies on a slavish pill-taking routine with little margin for error. It also has a higher failure rate in this age group: 4% at age 25 and probably considerably higher in the under-20s. However, Cerazette is a new POP (75 μg of desogestrel daily) designed to inhibit ovulation. A study comparing Cerazette with Microval showed that only 1.7% of cycles were ovulatory in Cerazette users, compared with 40% in Microval users (Rice *et al.* 1999). In a randomized trial of Cerazette versus Microval, the Pearl Index was 0.17 (method failure) and 0.5 (user failure) for Cerazette compared with 1.4 (method failure) and 1.9 (user failure) for Microval in non-breast-feeding women (Korver *et al.* 1998). Although the bleeding pattern in Cerazette users is more variable than with Microval, there is a greater tendency towards infrequent bleeding and amenorrhoea by the end of the first year. It would appear reasonable, in view of the ovulation inhibition, that there could be a 12-hour pill-taking safety margin rather than the three hours normally advised for conventional POPs (Korver *et al.* 2005). In June 2004 the Cerazette licence was revised to allow a 12-hour window for missed pills. Removal of the 'fear of forgetting' should make this POP a much more attractive option and improve compliance.

Withdrawal

A significant number of teenagers rely on this method in the early stages of their sexual experience. The failure rate is high, partly because teenage boys rarely have sufficient sexual control, and also because they are often simply unaware of the number of sperm in a single drop of semen. However, it is better than no method at all and has the advantage of always being available. Care should be taken not to discredit the method outright, since there is then a danger of teenagers feeling there is no point using it, even when they find themselves with no other option.

Rhythm method

A number of teenagers and indeed older women think they are using this method, when, in fact, they do not know when the 'safe period' is. The most common error is to consider the postmenstrual phase safe, allowing neither for the capriciousness of sperm survival nor the frequent occurrence of precocious ovulation. Even assuming they are informed, calculations and mucus observations are made difficult by the irregularity of the menstrual cycle in adolescence. Since, if used correctly, the method relies on lengthy abstinence, it is poorly suited to the unpredictable, opportunistic nature of teenage sexual activity.

The same applies to the Persona, which has the added disadvantage that it is not available on the NHS. It costs about £50 for the monitor and about £10 per month for the urine test sticks. When used absolutely correctly, with abstinence during the red days, the failure rate has been shown to be 6 per 100 woman-years. However, the user failure rate in the study was over 20 per 100 woman-years. In addition, the complicated instructions and requirement for up to 16 urine tests per cycle is likely to be too much for the average teenager.

Sterilization

This should only be considered in very exceptional circumstances, and then only as a team decision after a case conference. Carrying out a sterilization procedure for a mentally handicapped woman, especially if she is young, may legally constitute an assault. Great care should be taken to assess whether the woman is capable of giving informed consent. Indeed, a legal opinion (Mr Justice Woolf, 1983) has suggested that any person under the age of 16 is unlikely to be capable of consent to sterilization. In most circumstances, an injectable or an IUD will prove acceptable alternatives.

Emergency contraception

Emergency contraception is very important for teenagers. Over a quarter of teenagers use no contraception at all, and this is even more likely at the beginning of a relationship. It is therefore extremely important that they know about and have access to emergency contraception. Not only can it prevent an unwanted pregnancy, but it also gives an opportunity to discuss and initiate future long-term contraception. Many teenagers use the Family Planning service for the first time to obtain the emergency contraception.

Levonelle is both more effective than PC4 and has fewer side effects. And it can be obtained from pharmacies. More areas are now operating Patient Group Directives, so that women can obtain it free of charge from pharmacies. Otherwise it costs over £20 a time, which is likely to exclude many teenagers.

An IUD can, however, be fitted, in good faith, up to 5 days after the calculated date of ovulation, even after multiple exposures. This may sometimes be useful if the risk of conception seems high, but must be weighed against the trauma of insertion and the risk of infection (see above). Antibiotic cover and removal after the next period are relevant options to consider. In practice, most teenagers coming for post-coital contraception want the 'morning after Pill'.

Improving use of contraceptive services by young people

There is no doubt that young peoples' services are important in providing care for this group (Box 7.4). However, what is often forgotten is that most young people access services, such as general practice, that are generic and not age specific. As part of the process of developing services we must ensure that all relevant services are 'young people

Box 7.4 Improving teenagers' use of contraceptive services

- Ensure a range of services are available, both dedicated young people services and generic services that are young people friendly
- Advertise services
- Make access easy (timing, location, welcoming)
- Train staff (confidentiality, attitudes, etc.)
- Assure confidentiality (have a written policy)

friendly'. This means that they provide an environment that is welcoming, non-judgemental, accessible and is confidential and also perceived as being so.

Incidentally, much of what young people want from services is actually what all of us want. The difference is that we clearly need to increase use of services by young people if we are to achieve health benefit. There is debate about the provision services dedicated to young people with an upper age limit, usually 20 or 25, after which clients have to transfer to 'adult' services. Whilst definitely having a role, there are issues with this model; it sends a message to young people that generic services are not for them and also a message to the service that they do not need to cater for the needs of young people. Ensuring that all services providing sexual health care are young people friendly increases access to services and is acceptable to young people themselves.

What constitutes a young people friendly service?

The main components are: accessibility, non-judgemental staff, confidentiality, environment, wide range of services and information (about services and methods).

Accessibility

The location of most existing services is already set in stone; however, clinics that can be accessed easily by public transport yet are discreet are best for young poeple. Opening times that suit the lifestyles of young people are important, especially for younger teenagers who are still at school. The best time is late afternoon, so that they can 'drop in' on the way home or not 'too early' on a Saturday morning! A flexible system that combines appointments with a 'walk-in' facility offers the best access. This allows for the disorganized nature of many teenagers' lives, and also encourages teenagers who need, or feel they need, urgent advice. Since many teenagers lack motivation, it is important that neither the wait for an appointment, nor the actual waiting time in the clinic should be long.

Environment

Young people do not usually mind 'older people' being in the clinic, but they do like the place to appear as if they are meant to be there, and posters advertising services for them. A TV programme or magazines aimed at the younger person help to achieve this.

Services

Contraceptive advice, instant pregnancy testing, screening for sexually transmitted disease and, for those over 20, cervical smears, should all be core components to sexual health care for young people. This should include emergency contraception. However, some studies have shown that young people also like to be able to get health advice on other matters such as weight and skin problems. General practice is the most appropriate location to provide this wide provision of care.

Non-judgemental well informed staff

First impressions are important. All staff who come into contact with teenagers, including the reception staff, need to be aware of confidentiality and how to deal with their needs. Going to a new clinic can be intimidating even for grown ups and is often more so for younger clients. In the case of teenagers, a friendly, non-judgemental attitude is critical, as is sensitivity in realizing that the girl may need an urgent appointment for emergency contraception (Box 7.5).

A sexual health consultation with a young person may take longer than the average patient. They may not get around to saying what they want straight away. For example, 'I want to go on the Pill' may be used

Box 7.5 Improving teenagers' use of contraception

- Listen
- Teach condom use
- Explain availability of PCC
- Offer a range of methods
- Dispel myths/Discuss side effects
- Give instruction leaflets
- Early follow-up
- On-site pregnancy tests
- Don't forget STIs

as a general phrase for 'I want contraception', rather than specifically relating to the pill. They may want to discuss relationships, or non-contraceptive issues such as weight or acne. You need to make them feel you are interested in them as people not necessarily just an accident waiting to happen. You or the client may also have concerns about their risk for STI and this may need to be brought into the consultation.

If possible, teach all young people how to use a condom. Try to suggest the double Dutch method of pill plus condom. Most sexually active heterosexuals need to know about emergency contraception and this applies no less to young people. However, knowing about it also means knowing where to get it in a emergency. A consultation about emergency contraception needs to reinforce that they have behaved responsibly in coming and use the opportunity to advise on future contraception rather than being an excuse to chastise them for having unprotected sex. Comments such as 'I hope you won't need to use this again' may give the impression that you do not want to see the person again if they need emergency contraception and may indirectly lead to unplanned pregnancy.

Confidentiality

Confidentiality is of paramount importance, and equally important is that the teenagers understand that it exists. It is useful to have a written confidentiality policy or leaflet, such as the one produced by the Brook Advisory Clinics, that is visible to patients.

Information

Although the vast majority will use the pill or the condom, they, like other people, may want to know about other options. Particularly in the case of hormonal methods, check what they know and dispel any myths, which may cause trouble later. The same applies to side effects. Always give written information to back up what you've said. For teenagers, as with adults, the stress of the consultation is likely to mean they forget a lot of what they have been told. The FPA produce a good set of information leaflets for users. It may be useful to give the first follow-up appointment earlier than usual, to make sure they are happy and using the method correctly, particularly with the pill. Usually we would see new patients at 3 months, but an extra appointment at 6 weeks may be a good idea for teenagers.

Conclusion

It can be seen that in the area of teenage sexuality there are many issues and no easy solutions. One thing is clear: teenage sexual ill health is a fact and will not disappear if we pretend it does not exist. Much could be achieved if more adults with influence over young peoples' lives could acknowledge this and work together at finding practical solutions. It is a sobering thought that the observation made by Shakespeare over 300 years ago is still applicable to many teenagers today:

> For never was a story of more woe
> Than that of Juliet and her Romeo.

References and further reading

Barron SL. (1986) Sexual activity in girls under 16 years of age. *Br J Obstet Gynaecol* **93**, 787–93.

Blos P. (1972) The child analyst looks at the young adolescent. In: Kagan J, Coles R, (eds), *Twelve to sixteen: early adolescence.* New York: Norton.

Bury J. (1984) *Teenage pregnancy in Britain.* London: Birth Control Trust.

Bury J. (1986a) Teenagers and contraception. *Br J Fam Plann* **12**(1), 11–14.

Bury J. (1986b) Teenagers and contraception – II. *Br J Fam Plann* **12**(2), 42–7.

Cates W Jr, Schulz K, Grimes D. (1983) The risks associated with teenage abortion. *N Engl J Med* **309**, 6214.

Chilman C. (1979) *Adolescent sexuality in a changing American society. Social and psychological perspectives.* DHEW Publication No. 791426. Washington, DC: National Institutes of Health.

Faculty of Family Planning and Reproductive Health Care Clinical Effectiveness Unit FFPRHC Guidance (2004) Contraceptive choices for young people. *J Fam Plann Reprod Health Care* **30**(4), 237–51.

Ford N. (1992) The sexual and contraceptive lifestyles of young people: part 1. *Br J Fam Plann* **18**, 52–5.

Francome C. (1986) *Abortion practice in Britain and the United States.* London: Allen & Unwin.

Griffiths S. (1986) Providing care for sexually active adolescents. *Br J Fam Plann* **12**(3), 92–8.

Jones EF, Forrest JD, Goldman N *et al.* (1985) Teenage pregnancy in developed countries: determinants and policy implications. *Fam Plann Perspect* **17**(2), 53–63.

Korver T, Dieben T, Vree M, Van Muijen AE, Vromans L, Van Der Sanden A, Van Osta G. (1998) A double-blind study comparing the contraceptive efficacy, acceptability and safety of two progestogen-only pills containing desogestrel 75 micrograms/day or levonorgestrel 30 micrograms/day.

Collaborative Study Group on the Desogestrel-containing Progestogen-only Pill. *Eur J Contracept Reprod Health Care* **3**(4), 169–78.

Korver T, Klipping C, Heger-Mahn D, Duijkers I, van Osta G, Dieben T. (2005) Maintenance of ovulation inhibition with the 75-microg desogestrel-only contraceptive pill (Cerazette) after scheduled 12-h delays in tablet intake. *Contraception* **71**(1), 8–13.

Rice C, Killick SR, Dieben T, Coehlingh Bennink H. (1999) A comparison of the inhibition of ovulation achieved by desogestrel 75 mcg and levonorgestrel 30 mcg daily. *Hum Reprod* **14**(4), 982–5.

Rogstad KE, Ahmed-Jushuf IH, Robinson AJ. (2002) Standards for comprehensive sexual health services for young people under 25 years. *Int J STD AIDS* **13**, 420–4.

Rubinstein EA, Comstock GA, Murray JP. (Eds) (1972) *Television and social behavior, vol. IV: patterns of use.* Washingon, DC: Government Printing Office.

Simms M, Smith C. (1986) *Teenage mothers and their partners.* London: HMSO.

Skinner C. (1986) *Elusive Mr. Right.* London: Carolina Publications.

Trobisch W. (1972) *I married you.* London: Intervarsity Press.

Wellings K. (1986) Trends in contraceptive method usage since 1970. *Br J Fam Plann* **12**, 57–64.

Wellings K, Nanchahal K, Macdowall W *et al.* (2001) Sexual behaviour in Britain: early heterosexual experience. *Lancet* **358**, 1843–50.

Williams E. (1994) Contraceptive compliance among young people. *Br J Sex Med* **May/June**.

8 CONTRACEPTION FOR WOMEN OVER 40

It is often said that as fertility declines after the age of 35 the need for effective contraception also declines. However, women have been known to give birth after natural conception in their early 50s and thus the need for effective contraception must not be underestimated. Methods of contraception that at younger ages have unacceptably high failure rates may become a reasonable option in older women. Although it has been shown that coital frequency reduces with increasing age, new relationships are associated with an increase in coital frequency. This is relevant to many people in their 40s as long-term relationships end and new ones develop. Although the actual number of pregnancies in women over 40 is relatively small, a much higher proportion is likely to end in a termination, 37% compared to 23% for all ages (Office of National Statistics 1999). So although the risk of becoming pregnant is lower, because fertility declines with age, when a pregnancy does occur, there is a high chance it is unwanted, and may cause considerable distress.

Pregnancy in older women is not without risk. Spontaneous abortion rates, maternal mortality and perinatal mortality are all higher in women over 40, while the risk of Down's syndrome at the age of 40 is about 15 times what it was at the age of 20 (Table 8.1).

Table 8.1 Risk of Down's syndrome by age

Maternal age	Risk of trisomy
20–24	1 in 1500
25–29	1 in 1200
30–34	1 in 900
35–39	1 in 300
40–44	1 in 100
45+	1 in 40

Although the average age at menopause in this country is 51, many women start to get symptoms of oestrogen deficiency well before then (the perimenopause). Symptoms such as flushes, sleeplessness, depression and nervousness become increasingly common throughout the 40s, not just at the time of the menopause itself. The concept of a gradual reduction in menstruation leading up to the menopause is a myth, with many women experiencing irregular, painful and often heavier periods, rather than the reverse. This causes anxiety and may lead to gynaecological investigation, sometimes unnecessarily.

The features of the ideal contraceptive for this age group, if it were available, are shown in Box 8.1. The combined oral contraceptive pill (or the EVRA patch) would fulfil the majority of these criteria, but older women (and their doctors) are often reluctant to continue this method into the perimenopause. It is often forgotten that, although women who smoke must stop the pill at the age of 35, healthy, non-smoking women with no risk factors for vascular disease (with the exception of age) can take combined preparations until the age of 50.

Box 8.1 Desirable features of contraceptives for women over 40

- Acceptable efficacy
- Improves sex life. Ideally, the couple should not be worried that the method could fail. It should not be intercourse related, and should prevent vaginal dryness, which may occur in the perimenopause
- Control of climacteric symptoms: for example, flushes
- Control of 'normal' menstrual cycle (including heavy, irregular, painful periods)
- Decreased rate of gynaecological pathology, decreased risks of medical treatment and hysterectomy: for example, fibroids, endometriosis, cancers of older women such as ovarian and endometrial
- Protection against osteoporosis
- No masking of the menopause
- No systemic side effects, e.g. raised blood pressure, breast cancer

Combined oestrogen-progestogen contraceptives have many advantages for older women. In addition to a reduction in all problems associated with menstruation, an important benefit in this age group is an approximately 50% reduction in the risk of both ovarian and endometrial cancers. This protective effect continues for about 15 years after stopping the method. (See also Chapter 2)

The risk of breast cancer in oral contraceptive users has been the topic of a number of pill scares in the last 15 years (see also Chapter 2). A recent overview of 90% of the studies so far carried out (Collaborative Group on Hormonal Factors in Breast Cancer 1996) suggests a small increase in risk in having breast cancer diagnosed [relative risk (RR) 1.24] in women who are current users of combined oral contraceptives. This excess risk declines progressively after cessation of use, disappearing altogether after 10 years. There was no effect of pill dose or of duration of use, making a causal association unlikely. Breast cancers diagnosed in pill users were clinically less advanced than those in never-users, and were less likely to have spread beyond the breast. This would suggest that mortality from breast cancer might actually be reduced in pill users. It is possible that the pill accelerates the growth of tumours that were already present, thus making them clinically obvious earlier. A second possibility is that of surveillance bias; women who take the pill receive more medical attention and may be more 'breast aware'. Whilst in epidemiological terms this increased risk is small, given the frequency of breast cancer in women over 40 it would be prudent to ensure the patient is aware of these data and to consider other methods in women with a significant family history of breast cancer.

Reassuring evidence of the safety of the combined pill comes from the Royal College of General Practitioners' Study, which has recently published data on a 25-year follow-up of its cohort of 46 000 women (Beral *et al.* 1999). Most of the data relate to use of high-dose pills (50 μg and above of ethinylestradiol), but even these had no overall effect on mortality over the 25-year period. In addition, any effects of the pill ceased within 10 years of stopping the method.

Which pill for the older woman?

Third-generation pills were designed with the idea of reducing arterial disease risk, which may be more important in older women. They have fewer adverse effects on cholesterol and lipids, and also cause less insulin resistance than second-generation pills. Epidemiological evidence to confirm such a benefit has been difficult to obtain, with studies showing conflicting results. However, the most recent study (Tanis *et al.* 2001) showed an increased risk of myocardial infarction (RR 2.5) for women using second-generation pills, and no increase in risk for those on third-generation pills. In addition, the HDL Atherosclerosis Treatment Study (HATS) used a statin and niacin to raise HDL levels and showed regression of coronary artery disease (Brown *et al.* 2001). This major study at last provides clinical evidence to justify the previously only theoretical interest in oral contraceptive effects on HDL. It should, however, be reiterated that women over 35 with risk factors for arterial disease should not use oestrogen-containing contraceptives.

Obviously, older women on the pill should be carefully monitored to make sure, for example, that their blood pressure does not go up. This may be unrelated to their use of the pill, but would add a risk factor. If there were any suggestion of cardiovascular disease in a close relative under 50, it would be advisable to consider other methods and screen for lipid and clotting disorders.

With regard to the risk of venous thrombosis (VTE), older women are unlikely to be first-time users, so they should be a relatively low-risk group with regard to VTE (see also Chapter 9). Women with genetic disorders of clotting are more likely to have a VTE within a year of starting any type of combined pill. Thrombophilia screening is often carried out for those with a strong family history (a first-degree relative with VTE under the age of 45), but a negative result is not conclusive; even among women who have had a VTE, only about 50% will demonstrate a thrombophilia using the tests currently available. The risk of both arterial and venous disease goes up with age, so it is important to check for other risk factors for VTE. Recent studies have shown that a body mass index (BMI) of 35 or above carries a fourfold risk of VTE in women on the pill, while a BMI between 30 and 35 doubles the risk (Farmer *et al.* 2000; Jick *et al.* 2000). Women with a BMI over 30 would therefore be better advised to look at alternative, non-oestrogen containing methods (CSM 2004)

When to stop combined contraceptives

Combined preparations mask the menopause and the question therefore arises as to when to stop using contraception. It is necessary to use another method and stop the combined contraceptive at the age of 50 and do a follicle-stimulating hormone (FSH) level after a couple of months. If it is more than 30 IU/L, the woman can be considered menopausal. Conventionally, she should still use some other form of contraception for another year. Although it would not be possible to give an absolute guarantee of safety, some women may be reassured sufficiently to stop using all contraception. Of course, she may also choose to start using hormone replacement therapy (HRT).

Combined preparations for the future

In the near future, combined oestrogen-progestogen contraception will also be available in the form of a vaginal ring (NuvaRing) and possibly combined injectables. These are discussed in detail in Chapter 6.

Progestogen-only methods

So what about women who do not want to or can no longer use combined methods, for example because they smoke? All the progestogen-only methods can usually be considered by them until contraception is no longer required, irrespective of age.

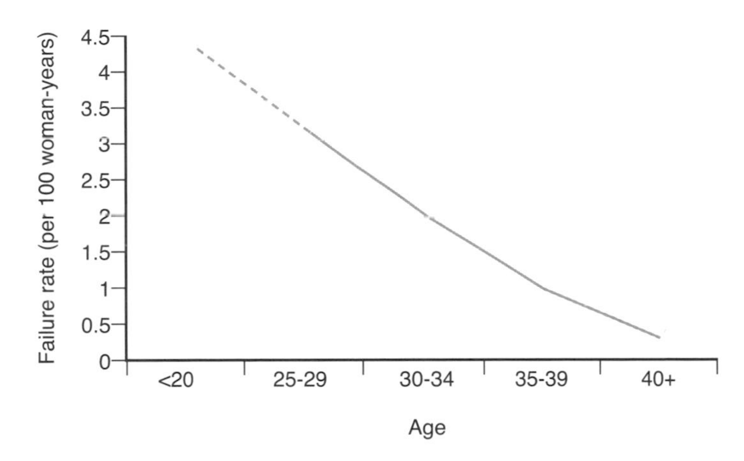

Figure 8.1 Graph of efficacy at different ages with POP. Source: Vessey MP, Lawless M, Yeates D, McPherson K. (1985) Progestogen only oral contraception. *Br J Fam Plann* **10**, 117–21.

The progestogen-only pill (POP) becomes a more attractive option as women get older. By the age of 40, the POP is as effective as the combined pill, and is already approaching this figure even at the age of 35 (see Figure 8.1). In addition, older women, who tend to lead more organized lives, may find it easier to cope with the rigid 3-hour rule, which is so important for this pill.

The potential problems associated with the POP are predominantly in relation to the effect on bleeding pattern. Irregular bleeding is a common side effect and in women over 40 may lead to further investigation, such as pelvic ultrasound or endometrial biopsy, which may not always be necessary. In addition, 15–20% of women on current POPs develop amenorrhoea, which may lead to anxiety about pregnancy.

A new addition is a 75 µg desogestrel POP, Cerazette, which reliably inhibits ovulation. As a result, women tend to bleed infrequently, and are more likely to become amenorrhoeic. In view of the ovulation inhibition, in June 2004 the Cerazette licence was revised to allow a 12-hour window for missed pills rather than the 3 hours normally advised for conventional POPs (Korver *et al.* 2005). Removal of the 'fear of forgetting' should make it a much more attractive option for many women.

The diagnosis of the menopause in an amenorrhoeic woman on the POP is simpler than with combined methods. POPs do not inhibit the production of FSH and measurements of this whilst still taking the POP are reliable. When a woman reaches 50, an FSH level should be done. If it is low, the POP (or another method) should be continued. However, if it is high, the procedure is the same as for women on the combined pill: they should stop the POP for 2 months and then the FSH level should be tested again. If it is still high, the woman is amenorrhoeic and has hot flushes, then she is almost certainly menopausal.

Depo-Provera

Progestogen can also be given in the form of long-acting injections such as Depo-Provera. This is an extremely effective contraceptive at all ages, with an overall failure rate of 0.1 per 100 woman-years. Like the POP, it can cause irregular bleeding, but is much more likely to result in amenorrhoea.

The effect of Depo-Provera on bone mineral density is discussed in detail elsewhere (see Chapter 3). However, in summary, women using this method should be assessed for other risk factors for osteoporosis and managed on the basis of this assessment. The measurement of serum oestradiol is not indicated on the basis of Depo-Provera use alone.

Depo-Provera could be a useful way of providing both contraception and HRT for older women. Depo-Provera has been shown to confer substantial protection against endometrial cancer, so all that is needed is to add oestradiol in whichever form the woman prefers. The result is a continuous combined, no-bleed HRT, which is popular with women who would like to continue using Depo-Provera in their 40s. This is an unlicensed indication, so should be done on a named-patient basis, but is becoming increasingly common practice.

Another useful progestogen-only method is Implanon, a single rod etonogestrel-releasing implant, which lasts for 3 years. Its hormone level is designed to achieve complete inhibition of ovulation and so far, in the worldwide phase III clinical trials, there has not been a single pregnancy. Both insertion and removal are considerably easier and quicker than was the case with older six-rod implant, Norplant, which is no longer available in the UK.

Amenorrhoea is more common in Implanon users than with Norplant (21% versus 10%, respectively). However, there is no evidence that hypo-oestrogenicity is a problem in Implanon users. Irregular bleeding can be a problem, as with all progestogen-only methods, and in the older age group may result in unnecessary investigation, as with the POP. However, at least pregnancy is not a worry for those women who become amenorrhoeic, since the method is more effective and there is no possibility of having forgotten a pill.

Summary of contraceptive use by older women

The main points for contraceptive use by older women are shown in Box 8.2.

Intrauterine methods

Copper intrauterine devices (IUDs) are often a very suitable method of contraception for the older woman. Whilst being very effective at all ages, the efficacy is greatest in the over-40s; thus if a women is older

Box 8.2 Points for contraceptive pill use by older women

- Healthy, non-smoking women can use oestrogen-containing contraceptives until age 50.
- Those who smoke, have a strong family history of arterial disease, or have a BMI over 30 can still use progestogen-only methods.
- All progestogen-only methods can cause irregular bleeding or amenorrhoea.
- POPs (other than Cerazette) are more effective in older women than in younger women.

than 40 when she has a copper IUD fitted, there is no need to change it, irrespective of the licence, and she can have it removed at an appropriate time after the menopause. Other positive aspects of IUD use in this age group include:

- the majority of such women are likely to have had a child, making the insertion easier;
- periods are often less painful after having a child, another advantage for a prospective IUD user;
- relationships are generally more stable, reducing the likelihood of infection.

However, there will be a subgroup of women older than 40 who are already experiencing heavier menstruation, which may become unacceptable after IUD insertion. For these women, the Mirena intrauterine system (IUS) may be a more appropriate method.

Mirena is a very acceptable method for many women older than 40, not just those with menorrhagia (Faculty of FP 2004). It is an intrauterine system releasing 20 µg of levonorgestrel per day and licensed for 5 years' use. However, when inserted in a woman aged 45 or over an IUS can be used off licence for 7 years, or, if she is amenorrhoeic, until contraception is no longer required (Faculty of FP 2004; NICE LARC 2005). Its mechanism of action is mainly related to atrophy of the endometrium, and the majority of women will ovulate at least occasionally after the first year of use. The failure rate of Mirena (0.2 per 100 woman-years) is comparable to sterilization and, unlike its proges-

Box 8.3 IUD use in older women

- A copper-containing IUD inserted after the age of 40 can provide acceptable contraception until after the menopause.
- The risks of pelvic infection after insertion of a copper IUD or Mirena are very low in this age group.
- Mirena reduces bleeding and may be an alternative to hysterectomy or sterilization.
- Mirena can provide both contraception and the progestogen part of HRT.

terone-releasing predecessor, is associated with a reduced risk of ectopic pregnancy when compared to no contraceptive use. In addition to being a very effective contraceptive, the IUS results in a major reduction in menstrual flow and dysmenorrhoea, making it a viable alternative to hysterectomy and endometrial ablation in women with menorrhagia (for which it now has a license). It does not appear to increase the risk of pelvic inflammatory disease. Irregular, though light, bleeding also occurs, particularly in the first few months of use. Only about 10–15% of women become amenorrhoeic.

The Mirena is proving invaluable for perimenopausal women who still need contraception, as it also provides the progestogen part of HRT. A licence for use (for 4 years) as the progestogen part of HRT was obtained in November 2004.

A summary of IUD use in older women is shown in Box 8.3.

Barrier methods and other alternatives

Barrier methods are quite suitable as the relatively high failure rates seen in young women are not a feature of use by well-motivated older women. Couples who have used them before are often quite happy to continue, but those who are unused to them sometimes find it quite a shock after the ease and spontaneity associated with, for instance, pill use. Some men may find it harder to maintain an erection when using the sheath. Women who have lax vaginal walls because of childbirth may find keeping a diaphragm in can be difficult although the arcing spring diaphragm or a cervical cap may be the answer.

Natural family planning, including Persona, is not generally suitable for this group of women because they tend to have irregular periods (with fluctuating hormone levels) and that makes any predictions very precarious.

Coitus interruptus may be more effective in older couples, especially if the man is experienced in its use. However, the failure rate is likely to remain higher than most of the alternatives until the woman is older than 45 years.

Emergency contraception

Even if a woman's fertility is deemed to be low, emergency contraception can be as important in preventing unplanned and unwanted pregnancy as in other age groups. Levonelle is a progestogen-only emergency pill, which is safe, has few side effects and provides significant reduction in the risk of pregnancy. Another advantage is its availability through pharmacists, which may be useful in this age group, who are more likely to be able to afford the £20 price. However, Levonelle does not provide ongoing contraception, which an emergency IUD does and should be considered by women requesting emergency contraception.

Sterilization

In this country, sterilization has become the most popular form of contraception for couples where the woman is over 35. However, requests for reversal of sterilization, which is not usually available on the NHS, are not infrequent. Vasectomy is very safe, remains the most effective method of contraception and should be considered where the man is sure he has completed his family. We now have a number of reversible methods, which are as effective as female sterilization and women should be counselled about all these alternatives and have access to them before deciding on sterilization. In addition, a recent American review found a cumulative failure rate over a 10-year period of 18.5 per 1000 woman-years (Peterson *et al.* 1996). It should be noted that in the UK the Filshie clip is most commonly used (in contrast to the USA), and is thought to be more effective than most other procedures. In the UK, it is usual to quote the risk of lifetime failure as being 1 in 200, although data on the Filshie clip suggest a failure rate after 10 years of two to three per 1000 procedures (RCOG 2004). It is impor-

Box 8.4 Barrier methods and other alternatives

- Barrier methods are more effective in older couples.
- Natural family planning is not suitable for women with irregular periods.
- Emergency contraception should not be forgotten.
- Counselling about reversible alternatives is important for couples considering sterilization.

tant that the woman has a gynaecological history and examination, even if it is her partner who is considering a vasectomy. She may sometimes have a gynaecological problem for which she should consider a hysterectomy, rendering any sterilization unnecessary.

Counselling also needs to take into account that the years around the menopause are a time of many psychological problems for both men and women. These can actually be made worse by the very finality of sterilization.

Box 8.4 lists the various points regarding barrier methods and other alternatives for the older woman.

References and further reading

Beral V, Hermon C, Kay C, Hannaford P, Darby S, Reeves G. (1999) Mortality associated with oral contraceptive use: 25 year follow up of cohort of 46,000 women from the Royal College of General Practitioners' oral contraception study. *Br Med J* **318**, 96–100.

Brown BG, Zhao XQ, Chait A *et al.* (2001) Simvastatin and niacin, antioxidant vitamins, or the combination for the prevention of coronary disease. *N Engl J Med* **345**, 1583–92.

Collaborative Group on Hormonal Factors in Breast Cancer (1996) Breast cancer and hormonal contraceptives: collaborative reanalysis of individual data of 53,297 women with breast cancer and 100,239 women without breast cancer from 54 epidemiological studies. *Lancet* **347**, 1713–27.

Committee on the Safety of Medicines (2004) Combined oral contraceptives: venous thromboembolism. *Current Problems in Pharmacovigilance* **30**, 7.

Faculty of Family Planning and Reproductive Health Care Clinical Effectiveness Unit. FFPRHC Guidance (2004) The levonorgestrel-releasing intrauterine system (LNG-IUS) in contraception and reproductive health. *J Fam Plann Reprod Health Care* **30**(2), 99–109.

Faculty of Family Planning and Reproductive Health Care Clinical Effectiveness Unit. FFPRHC Guidance (2005) Contraception for women aged over 40 years. *J Fam Plann Reprod Health Care* **31**(1), 51–64.

Farmer RDT, Lawrenson RA, Todd JC *et al.* (2000) A comparison of the risks of venous thromboembolic disease in association with different combined oral contraceptives. *Br J Clin Pharmacol* **49**, 580–90.

Gbolade BA. (2002) Depo-Provera and bone density. *J Fam Plann Reprod Health Care* **28**(1), 7–11.

Jick H, Kaye JA, Vasilakis-Scaramozza C, Jick SS. (2000) Risk of venous thromboembolism among users of third generation oral contraceptives compared with users of oral contraceptives with levonorgestrel before and after 1995: cohort and case-control analysis. *Br Med J* **321**, 1190–5.

Korver T, Klipping C, Heger-Mahn D, Duijkers I, van Osta G, Dieben T. (2005) Maintenance of ovulation inhibition with the 75-microg desogestrel-only contraceptive pill (Cerazette) after scheduled 12-h delays in tablet intake. *Contraception* **71**(1), 8–13.

NICE LARC guideline (2005) *Long-acting reversible contraception: the effective and appropriate use of long-acting reversible contraception.* London: National Institute for Health and Clinical Excellence.

Peterson HB, Xia Z, Hughes JM, Wilcox LS, Tylor LR, Trussell J. (1996) The risk of pregnancy after tubal sterilization: findings from the US Collaborative Review of Sterilization (CREST). *Am J Obstet Gynecol* **174**, 1161–70.

Royal College of Obstetricians and Gynaecologists (2004) *Male and female sterilisation: evidence-based clinical guideline* Number 4. London: RCOG Press.

Szarewski A, Guillebaud J. (2002) *Contraception: a user's handbook,* 3rd edition. Oxford: Oxford University Press.

Tanis BC, van den Bosch MAAJ, Kemmeren JM *et al.* (2001) Oral contraceptives and the risk of myocardial infarction. *N Engl J Med* **345**(25), 1787–93.

Vessey MP, Lawless M, Yeates D, McPherson K. (1985) Progestogen only oral contraception. *Br J Fam Plann* **10**, 117–21.

9 CONTRACEPTION FOR WOMEN AT RISK OF VENOUS THROMBOEMBOLISM

The term venous thromboembolism (VTE) comprises deep vein thrombosis (DVT) of the legs and pelvis, pulmonary embolism (PE) and cerebral sinus thrombosis (CST). The incidence of VTE rises with age, from one per 100 000 people per year in childhood to nearly 1% per year in old age (Rosendaal 1999). Looking specifically at DVT in women aged 15–49 years, it has been estimated that the overall incidence is 21 per 100 000 women per year (Vandenbroucke *et al.* 1996). In pregnancy, the risk of antenatal DVT is about 61 per 100 000 in women under the age of 35 and 121 per 100 000 in women over that age. The rate of postpartum DVT is about 30 per 100 000 in women under the age of 35 and 72 per 100 000 in older women (Greer 1999). Of those who suffer a DVT, about 1% will die, usually due to a pulmonary embolism.

Risk factors for venous thromboembolism

Venous thrombosis results from a combination of inherited and acquired risk factors (see Table 9.1).

Table 9.1 Risk factors for venous thromboembolism

Inherited	Acquired
Antithrombin deficiency	Immobility
Protein C deficiency	Surgery, trauma
Protein S deficiency	Obesity
Activated protein C resistance, factor V Leiden mutation	Pregnancy/puerperium
Factor XII deficiency	Long distance travel
	Use of combined oral contraceptives/ hormone replacement therapy
	Antiphospholipid antibody, lupus anticoagulant
	Malignancy

As more inherited thrombophilic conditions are identified, the role of inherited thrombophilias has been increasingly recognized during the last decade. It is now possible to identify a genetic contribution in approximately half the patients who present with a first DVT, and new genetic coagulation disorders are being discovered all the time. The coagulation system is constantly balancing the effects of procoagulants and anticoagulants. The major anticoagulant factors are:

- antithrombin, which neutralizes thrombin and other procoagulant enzymes;
- protein C, which inactivates cofactors V and VIII;
- protein S, the cofactor for protein C;
- thrombomodulin, which enables thrombin to activate protein C.

The classic thrombophilias are the ones arising from a deficiency of antithrombin, protein C or protein S. These cause an estimated 20-fold increase in the risk of thrombosis, but in absolute terms are rare, accounting for no more than 8% of patients investigated after a first thrombosis (Laffan and Tuddenham 1998).

However, the major breakthrough in this area was the discovery of factor V Leiden mutation in 1994 (Bertina *et al.* 1994). The mutated form of factor V is resistant to inactivation by protein C; since protein C is an anticoagulant (see above), the result is an increased tendency to thrombosis. This scenario is known as activated protein C (APC) resistance. Factor V Leiden is found in approximately 5% of Caucasians, though higher rates (15%) have been found in some populations, for example in Sweden and Greece (Vandenbroucke *et al.* 1996). However, the prevalence appears to be extremely low in African and Oriental women. The mutation is found in 20% of patients with VTE; among carriers, the risk of thrombosis is 57 per 100 000 women per year.

Since the discovery of factor V Leiden, several other genetic mutations have come to light, including another factor V variant (factor V Cambridge) and a prothrombin gene mutation (prothrombin 20210A), which was found in 18% of patients who had suffered a VTE (Provan and O'Shaughnessy 1999) but in only 12% of normal control subjects.

More complex genetic changes can result in abnormally high levels of clotting factors. This has been shown to be the explanation for the relatively increased risk of thrombosis in people with blood groups other than O, who have higher levels of clotting factor VIII. Factor VIII concentrations that exceed 1500 IU/L (150% of normal) have been found in 11% of the general population and 25% of patients with thrombosis. Such high concentrations were associated with a sixfold increase in the risk of thrombosis. Another example is that of hyperhomocysteinuria, whose sufferers have an increased risk (three- to fourfold) of thrombosis (Rosendaal 1999).

However, it is important to remember that one inherited defect of coagulation is unlikely to result in a VTE on its own. It is frequently found that individuals with thrombophilia have several genetic coagulation defects at the same time, and even then they are likely to require another, acquired risk factor, before thrombosis occurs.

Acquired risk factors, such as pregnancy, immobilization and use of combined oral contraceptives (COCs) are common. It is also often forgotten that increasing age is in itself a risk factor for thrombosis, and this is unavoidable. A feature that is common to thrombophilic families is that the mean age at first thrombosis is much younger than for consecutive patients with thrombosis, irrespective of the underlying defect and even when no defect has been identified (Table 9.2).

A synergistic effect has been shown for factor V Leiden and COC use. Women who use COCs but are not carriers of factor V Leiden have a risk of VTE of around 30 per 100 000 per year. The risk for carriers of the defect who do not use COCs is 57 per 100 000 per year. However, for women who are carriers and use COCs, the risk jumps to 285 per 100 000 per year (Vandenbroucke *et al.* 1996).

Similarly, COC use and the presence of thrombophilic coagulation defects lead to much higher risks of cerebral sinus thrombosis (30–150 times) than found in women who use COCs but do not have a thrombophilia (de Bruijn *et al.* 1998; Martinelli *et al.* 1998).

Table 9.2 Age at first thrombosis by origin of patient

Risk factor	Age (years) at first thrombosis	
	Patients from thrombophilic families (*n* = 78)	Consecutive unselected patients (*n* = 105)
Protein C deficiency	31	47
Factor V Leiden	29	43
No defect found	34	46

From Rosendaal FR (1999).

The combined oral contraceptive pill and venous thrombosis

The first definite link between the combined pill and venous thrombosis was made by the Royal College of General Practitioners (1967) Study and that of Vessey and Doll in 1968. At the time, the risk of VTE with these high-dose pills was estimated at 100 per 100 000 women per year (Vessey 1989). The risk of VTE was found to be dependent on the dose of oestrogen in the pill (Inman *et al.* 1970), and this was subsequently reduced. Studies which later looked at the risk of VTE with second-generation (30–35 mg ethinylestradiol) pills found risks of 39 and 42 per 100 000 women per year (Stadel 1981; Vessey *et al.* 1986; Gerstman *et al.* 1991).

In October 1995, the United Kingdom Committee on Safety of Medicines (CSM) released a 'Dear Doctor' letter, warning doctors about an increased risk of venous thromboembolism in women taking third-generation COC pills. These pills, containing the progestogens desogestrel and gestodene, had been on the market since the mid-1980s and were extremely popular. It has been estimated that in 1995 approximately 1.5 million women in the UK were taking this type of pill.

The papers on which the CSM based their advice were not published until later that year and the next year (Jick *et al.* 1995; WHO Collaborative Study of Cardiovascular Disease and Steroid Hormone Contraception 1995; Spitzer *et al.* 1996), resulting in considerable confusion. This was the first time that it had been suggested that a difference in progestogen type could so greatly influence venous thromboembolic risk, which had previously always been attributed to oestrogen.

The new studies showed a risk of VTE for users of third-generation pills of 30 per 100 000 women per year, which is in fact a slightly lower figure than that shown in previous studies for second-generation pills. However, in these studies the risk for second-generation pills had dropped to 15 per 100 000 women per year. The CSM therefore stated that there was a doubling of risk for users of third-generation pills and advised doctors that desogestrel- and gestodene-containing pills should no longer routinely be used as first-choice contraceptives.

Many doctors believe that regulatory action was unnecessary in 1995, and that the way in which it was carried out, prior to publication of the studies, was irresponsible (Edwards *et al.* 1997; Spitzer 1997, 1998; Benagiano 1998; Cohen 1998; Mills and Edwards 1999). None of the studies was beyond criticism and there has been much debate about the role of prescribing bias and confounding factors as possible explanations for the apparent increase in risk for third-generation pills.

The most obvious example of prescriber bias can be seen with the Mercilon/Marvelon paradox. Mercilon and Marvelon both contain the same amount (150 μg) of desogestrel, but in Marvelon this is combined with 30 μg ethinylestradiol, while in Mercilon the oestrogen dose is lower, at 20 μg. It would therefore seem self-evident that the risk of VTE should be lower in users of Mercilon, and yet in all the recent studies, risks for VTE have been higher in users of Mercilon. Clearly, doctors were prescribing the lower-dose product to women considered at higher risk (e.g. because of family history or obesity). This whole issue has been well summarized by Spitzer (1997).

The combined pill and VTE

There have been three new studies from the UK published in the last few years (Farmer *et al.* 2000a, b; Jick *et al.* 2000). All are based on the General Practice Research Database (GPRD).

The data published in the British Medical Journal in 2000 (Farmer *et al.* 2000b) showed that, contrary to expectation, there has been no change in the incidence of VTE since the 1995 pill scare. Between November 1995 and December 1998, the percentage of COCs prescribed containing either gestodene or desogestrel fell from 53.4% to 14%. If second-generation pills really are safer, one would have expected the VTE rates to be lower after the pill scare than before (especially considering doctors were now more aware of other risk factors). However, when VTE rates from the 2 years leading up to the scare were compared with the data after November 1995, no difference was found (34 versus 36 cases per 100 000 women per year).

The second study (Farmer *et al.* 2000a) is a nested case–control study, looking at VTE rates in second- and third-generation pill users. An overall incidence of 38 per 100 000 women per year was found (compatible with the incidence study) and no significant difference was found between the types of pills. Several interesting pieces of information have emerged from this study. A body mass index (BMI) of 35 or above carries a fourfold risk of VTE, while a BMI between 30 and 35 doubles the risk. Obesity is therefore a very important risk factor for VTE in women on the pill.

Smoking is a well-established risk factor for arterial disease, but in this study it also appears to be significant in VTE, resulting in a doubling of the risk. Interestingly, similar results regarding smoking and BMI were shown in the study by Jick *et al.* (2000), despite contrasting findings regarding VTE rates. For women with a BMI over 25, Jick found a sixfold increase in risk, and, like Farmer, a doubling of risk in smokers. Since then, there has been another study, from Denmark, showing a doubling of risk for women with a BMI over 25 and a fivefold increase in risk for women with a BMI over 30. This study also showed a doubling of risk for smokers, with a dose–response relationship.

This throws up further possibilities for prescriber bias: third-generation pills were actually marketed as potentially safer for use in women with arterial risk factors, such as smoking. If smoking is also a risk factor for VTE, and most women who smoke were preferentially given third-generation pills, that doubling of risk due to smoking could have contributed to an apparent increase in VTE associated with third-generation pills. Clearly, further studies need to be done, but there are already several previous studies showing a trend in this direction.

In 1998 the Department of Health announced an end to the 1995 restrictions on prescribing third-generation pills, stating that 'the absolute risk of VTE in women taking third-generation COCs is very small and is much less than the risk in pregnancy' and 'provided women are fully informed of these very small risks and do not have medical contraindications, it should be a matter of clinical judgement and personal choice which type of oral contraceptive should be prescribed' (Medicines Control Agency 1999). The effect of this was that third-generation pills could be prescribed as first-line again. In addition, in 2002, the Honourable Mr Justice Mackay handed down his judgment in the group action against the manufacturers of third-generation combined pills [EWHC 1420 (QB) 2002]. His conclusion was that:

> I find that there is not as a matter of probability any increased relative risk of VTE carried by any of the third generation oral contraceptives supplied to these Claimants by the Defendants as compared with second generation products containing Levonorgestrel. (para 339).

Recent data (the EURAS study) suggest no difference in VTE rates between second/third-generation pills, or Yasmin (Heinemann 2004). The same study suggests that all VTE rates (including those in pregnancy) are higher than previously thought: those for the COC are between 60 and 73 per 100 000 women-years, while the risk in pregnancy reaches as high as 800 per 100 000 women-years.

We should also be much more careful about BMI (CSM 2004). Ten years ago, there were fewer alternatives to the pill. However, we now have several highly effective and safe progestogen-only methods, which do not increase the risk of VTE. A BMI of 39 is an absolute contraindication to the COC, however alternative non-oestrogen containing methods should be recommended to all women with a BMI over 30 (CSM 2004) since this is associated with at least a fourfold increased risk of VTE. When Mirena, DMPA, IUDs, Implanon and the POP are available, prescribing the COC to women with a BMI over 30 should be unusual and, for a BMI over 35, rare (Szarewski 2000).

Benefits of third-generation pills

There is some evidence that third-generation COCs may be safer for women at risk of arterial disease, which would add another layer to the risk–benefit analysis, since, as mentioned above, some risk factors (now including smoking) for both arterial and venous disease overlap. The Transnational study (Lewis *et al.* 1997) has shown a statistically significant reduction in risk of myocardial infarction (MI) in users of desogestrel- and gestodene-containing pills, compared with second-generation products. The MICA study failed to show a difference between the two types of pill (Dunn *et al.* 1999). However, the most recent study (Tanis *et al.* 2001) showed a significantly increased risk of MI [relative risk (RR) 2.5] for women using second-generation pills, and no increase in risk for those on third-generation pills. In addition, the HDL Atherosclerosis Treatment Study (HATS) used a statin and niacin to raise HDL levels and showed regression of coronary artery disease (Brown *et al.* 2001). This major study at last provides clinical evidence to justify the previously only theoretical interest in oral contraceptive effects on HDL.

Third-generation pills have benefits in terms of quality of life, but this aspect is, unfortunately, difficult to quantify. Third-generation progestogens, while still giving good cycle control, are less androgenic than second-generation products and therefore tend to be better for women who have problems with acne, hirsutism, and weight gain (Szarewski and Mansour 1999).

Prescribing implications

Women who have already had an episode of VTE should not be prescribed oestrogen-containing contraceptives of any kind (Mills *et al.* 1998). The question has been raised as to whether all women considering the COC should be screened for thrombophilias. The answer is an unequivocal 'no'. It has been estimated that screening one million women would prevent one death per year from VTE (Mills *et al.* 1998). However, there is considerable debate around the issue of women who have a family history of VTE. Although, again, relatively few lives may be saved (four women per million screened), there is a consensus that this may occasionally be worthwhile for the individual. There are two main issues to consider. The first is if the screen is negative, these women still have an increased risk of VTE in comparison to women with no family history of VTE. The other issue is that of women who are found to have a thrombophilia, many will never have a VTE, but their future medical care, including in pregnancy, may be affected by the positive diagnosis, leading to unnecessary intervention.

What constitutes a family history? The strongest case can be made for a definite (proven) history of VTE in a first-degree relative under the age of 45. However, since women who are about to take the pill for the first time are likely to be young, their first-degree relatives may well not yet have had their VTE, the risk of which increases with age. Also, with family size becoming smaller, they may not have siblings at all. Stretching the criteria to include more distant relatives will certainly detect more cases, but at the cost of worrying a large number of women unnecessarily. A major problem with screening is that currently, even in people who have had a VTE, a coagulation defect can only be detected in about 50% (Hampton and Preston 1997). This means that a negative screen does not give complete reassurance: only a few years ago, all the women now known to be positive for factor V Leiden, with their greatly increased risk, would have been told they were 'clear'. This situation is likely to improve in the future, as more coagulation defects are recognized and the tests become simpler (and therefore cheaper to do 'en masse').

It is clear that screening for only one coagulation defect is not very useful: if screening is to be done at all, a bank of tests is required. The tests done will vary between laboratories; however, it would be usual to include assays of fibrinogen, antithrombin III, protein C, protein S, APC resistance, antiphospholipid antibodies, factor V Leiden mutation and prothrombin mutation (Machin *et al.* 1995). Some laboratories also carry out homocysteine levels. It seems to be a general principle in haemostatic screening that more (tests) is better. If all these tests are negative, the woman should still be advised that a thrombophilia cannot be absolutely excluded and that her risk of VTE is higher than for a woman with no family history, but, on this understanding, if she wishes to take the COC, it can be prescribed. However, it should not be forgotten that the reverse scenario is also true: many women found to have a thrombophilia will not in fact go on to develop a VTE and will therefore have been worried and may have avoided the pill unnecessarily. It should also be borne in mind that the greatest risk of VTE occurs in the first year of pill use (Spitzer 1997); thus, if a woman has already been on the pill for over a year (without having developed a VTE), she is likely to be at reduced risk.

Other risk factors and the COC

Since VTE is a multifactorial problem, even women without a family history may have risk factors which make taking the combined pill inadvisable. One of the most important of these is obesity, specifically a body mass index (BMI) of over 30 kg/m^2, as mentioned above. It is often assumed that women with varicose veins should be cautious about taking the pill, but this is not substantiated (Campbell 1996). However, women should be reminded to stop taking the pill about 4 weeks prior to major surgery or immobilization and not to resume for the same length of time afterwards (Guillebaud 1989).

Should first-time users and women with a family history of VTE (and negative screen) be prescribed second- or third-generation pills as first choice?

Since the revision of the 1995 CSM guidelines and the recent CSM statement (CSM 2004), this is now a matter for the prescriber and the individual woman, based on the risks and benefits of a particular pill in her case. The most recent data suggest that there is no difference in VTE risk between different pills (see above).

What about Dianette?

Dianette is in fact licensed as a treatment for acne and hirsutism, rather than a contraceptive, although it is also an effective contraceptive

(Aydinlik *et al.* 1990). The prescribing of Dianette for women judged to have polycystic ovary syndrome (PCOS) has steadily increased since 1992 (Seaman 2003), particularly in older women (over 25, but especially over 30).

Women with PCOS are likely to have an increased risk of cardiovascular disease (Laurel *et al.* 2002). They are more likely to be obese, have insulin resistance, dyslipidaemia and hypertension than women without PCOS. In the context of VTE risk, the obesity is likely to be the greatest problem, since, as discussed above, this is an important risk factor for VTE. Although some studies have suggested an increased risk of VTE in women on Dianette, it is unlikely that they have been able to control adequately for the effects of prescriber bias and confounding by these other risk factors (Seaman 2003).

Generally, Dianette is recommended for use as long as the acne or hirsutism persist: there are data on up to 5 years of use, which have suggested that in most women it should be possible to change to another brand after between 1 and 3 years, but if symptoms are still a problem, it may be continued for longer (Falsetti 2001). It is suggested that Dianette is stopped about 4 months after symptoms have resolved. Whenever the decision to stop is taken, it would then be logical to change to Marvelon, Cilest, or Yasmin. The randomized trials (Foidart *et al.* 2000; Huber 2000) comparing Yasmin with Marvelon showed that both pills were equally beneficial for acne. A randomized, double-blind trial of 125 women comparing Yasmin with Dianette showed that Yasmin was as effective as Dianette for women with mild to moderate acne (Van Vloten *et al.* 2002).

Other contraceptive options

If the woman cannot, or does not wish to use the combined pill, there are still many options open to her. However, it should be remembered that pregnancy also poses a very significant risk of VTE, and therefore the method chosen should preferably be very effective at preventing pregnancy.

Progestogen-only methods are all suitable for women at risk of VTE, as progestogen on its own has not been demonstrated to have any significant effects on coagulation. Nor has it been associated with VTE in epidemiological studies (Fotherby 1989a, b; Machin *et al.* 1995). Progestogen-only pills (Fotherby 1989a, b), injectable progestogens (Lande 1995), implants

(Machin *et al.* 1995; Egberg *et al.* 1998) and the intrauterine levonorgestrel-releasing system (Luukkainen 1991) are all possible choices. Of these, second-generation POPs are somewhat less effective in young women (Fotherby 1989a, b), with failure rates of around 4 per 100 woman-years. By the age of 35, however, efficacy is equivalent to that of the combined pill, at less than one per 100 woman-years.

Cerazette is a new desogestrel POP. The dose is 75 μg of desogestrel daily and it has been designed to inhibit ovulation. A study comparing Cerazette with Microval showed that only 1.7% of cycles were ovulatory in Cerazette users, compared to 40% in Microval users (Rice *et al.* 1999). In a randomized trial of Cerazette versus Microval, the Pearl Index was 0.17 (method failure) and 0.5 (user failure) for Cerazette compared with 1.4 (method failure) and 1.9 (user failure) for Microval in non-breast-feeding women (Korver *et al.* 1998). Although the bleeding pattern in Cerazette users is more variable than with Microval, there is a greater tendency towards infrequent bleeding and amenorrhoea by the end of the first year. In view of the ovulation inhibition, in June 2004 the Cerazette licence was revised to allow a 12-hour window for missed pills, rather than the 3 hours normally advised for conventional POPs (Korver *et al.* 2005). Removal of the 'fear of forgetting' should make it a much more attractive option for many women.

Doubling the daily dose of conventional POPs has been suggested as a policy in women who weigh more than 70 kg, and indeed is mentioned in the Family Planning Association (FPA) leaflet on POPs. There is, however, no evidence relating to the POP itself to suggest that there is indeed an increased failure rate in overweight women (Vessey 2001). What evidence exists relates to a progestogen-only vaginal ring (which was not marketed) and an early version of Norplant; for both these devices, the failure rate was two to four times higher in women weighing 70 kg. However, in the case of Norplant, a change in the density of the polymer was enough to deal with the problem, so the marketed version was not significantly affected by weight. The efficacy of Implanon also does not appear to be affected by weight. Thus, there seems little justification for such a policy for the POP. However, in the case of young women using conventional POPs, it might be reasonable to err on the side of caution in view of the already higher failure rate. It would appear that this will not be necessary with Cerazette, since blood levels, as with Implanon, are high enough to withstand any effect of increased weight.

All the other progestogen-only methods have very low failure rates (less than one per 100 woman-years) and have the advantage that they are all long-acting, requiring little effort on the part of the user. However, all (including the POP) have the side effect of causing irregularity of menstruation. Depomedroxyprogesterone acetate has a particular advantage in women with sickle cell disease (with its higher risk of thrombosis), as it has been shown to reduce the number of crises and improve the haematological picture (Lande 1995). Progestogen-only emergency contraception (Levonelle) is also safe for use in these women (WHO 1998).

Non-hormonal methods

All the non-hormonal methods are theoretically suitable, although barrier methods and natural family planning may have unacceptably high failure rates. Modern copper intrauterine devices (e.g. the T-Safe CU 380 A, the GyneFix) are extremely effective, with failure rates of less than one per 100 woman-years.

Conclusion

Women at risk of venous thrombosis have a wider choice of contraceptive methods than they (and their doctors) often think. History taking is important in order to elucidate familial risk as well as other potential risk factors. It should be remembered that VTE is a multifactorial disease, usually the result of an interaction between several risk factors, both genetic and acquired. In the future, screening for thrombophilia should become a better predictor of risk, as more coagulation defects are discovered and tests become simpler, cheaper and more comprehensive. In the interim, women at risk are in particular need of information to enable them to make what are often difficult decisions.

References and further reading

Aydinlik S, Kaufman J, Lochnit-Fixson U, Lehnert J. (1990) Long-term therapy of signs of androgenisation with a low dosed antiandrogen-oestrogen combination. *Clin Trials J* **27**(6), 392–402.

Benagiano G. (1998) Venous thromboembolism and the pill. Learning from the past, venous thromboembolism and the pill: an endless saga. *Hum Reprod* **13**(5), 1115–16.

Bertina RM, Koeleman BP, Koster T *et al.* (1994) Mutation in blood coagulation factor V associated with resistance to activated protein C. *Nature* **369**, 64–7.

Broome M, Macaulay O. (1996) Consider the progestogen-only pill. *Br J Fam Plann* **22**, 111.

Brown BG, Zhao XQ, Chait A *et al.* (2001) Simvastatin and niacin, antioxidant vitamins, or the combination for the prevention of coronary disease. *N Engl J Med* **345**, 1583–92.

Campbell B. (1996) Thrombosis, phlebitis and varicose veins. *Br Med J* **312**, 198–9.

Cohen J. (1998) Recommendations on the safety of oral contraceptives are too important for the regulating agencies alone. *Hum Reprod* **13**(5), 1116–17.

Committee on Safety of Medicines. (1995) *Combined oral contraceptives and thromboembolism.* London: CSM.

Committee on Safety of Medicines (2004) Combined oral contraceptives: venous thromboembolism. *Curr Prob Pharmacovigilance* **30**, 7.

CPMP position statement on oral contraceptives containing desogestrel or gestodene. CPMP/374/96. 17th April 1996.

Davies GC, Newton JR. (1991) Subdermal contraceptive implants – a review: with special reference to Norplant. *Br J Fam Plann* **17**, 4–8.

de Bruijn SFTM, Stam J, Koopman mmW, Vandenbroucke JP. (1998) Case-control study of risk of cerebral sinus thrombosis in oral contraceptive users who are carriers of hereditary prothrombotic conditions. *Br Med J* **316**, 589–92.

Department of Health. (1999) Oral contraceptives – clearer information for woman and health professionals. Press Release 07.04.99.

Dunn N, Thorogood M, Faragher B *et al.* (1999) Oral contraceptives and myocardial infarction: results of the MICA case-control study. *Br Med J* **318**, 1579–84.

Edwards RG, Beard HK, Bradshaw JP. (1997) Balancing risks and benefits of oral contraception. [editorial] *Hum Reprod* **12**(11), 2339–40.

Egberg N, van Beek A, Gunnervik C *et al.* (1998) Effects on the hemostatic system and liver function in relation to Implanon and Norplant. *Contraception* **58**, 93–8.

Falsetti L, Gambera A, Tisi G. (2001) Efficacy of the combination ethinyl-oestradiol and cyproterone acetate on endocrine, clinical and ultrasonographic profile in polycystic ovarian syndrome. *Hum Reprod* **16**(1), 36–42.

Farmer RDT, Lawrenson RA, Thompson CR, Kennedy JG, Hambleton IR. (1997) Population-based study of risk of venous thromboembolism associated with various oral contraceptives. *Lancet* **349**, 83–8.

Farmer RDT, Lawrenson RA, Todd JC *et al.* (2000a) A comparison of the risks of venous thromboembolic disease in association with different combined oral contraceptives. *Br J Clin Pharmacol* **49**, 580–90.

Farmer RDT, Williams TJ, Simpson EL, Nightingale AL. (2000b) The effect of the 1995 pill scare on rates of venous thromboembolism among women taking combined oral contraceptives: analysis of General Practice Research Database. *Br Med J* **321**, 477–9.

Foidart J-M, Wuttke W, Bouw GM, Gertlinger C, Heithecker R. (2000) A comparative investigation of contraceptive reliability, cycle control and tolerance of two monophasic oral contraceptives containing either drospirenone or desogestrel. *Eur J Contracept Reprod Health* **5**(2), 124 –34.

Fotherby K. (1989a) The progestogen-only pill and thrombosis. *Br J Fam Plann* **15**, 83–5.

Fotherby K. (1989b) The progestogen-only pill. In: Filshie M, Guillebaud J (eds), *Contraception: science and practice.* London: Butterworth, pp. 94–108.

Gerstman BB, Piper JM, Tomita DK, Ferguson WJ, Stadel BV, Lundin FE. (1991) Oral contraceptive estrogen dose and the risk of deep venous thromboembolic disease. *Am J Epidemiol* **133**, 32–7.

Greer IA. (1999) Thrombosis in pregnancy: maternal and fetal issues. *Lancet* **353**, 1258–65.

Guillebaud J. (1989) Practical prescribing of the combined oral contraceptive pill. In: Filshie M, Guillebaud J (eds), *Contraception: science and practice.* London: Butterworth, pp. 69–94.

Guillebaud J. (1995) Advising women on which pill to take. *Br Med J* **331**, 1111–12.

Hampton KK, Preston FE. (1997) Bleeding disorders, thrombosis and anticoagulation. *Br Med J* **314**, 1026–9.

Heinemann LAJ, Dinger J. (2004) Safety of a new oral contraceptive containing drospirenone. *Drug Safety* **27**(13), 1001–18.

Huber J, Foidart J-M, Wuttke W *et al.* (2000) Efficacy and tolerability of a monophasic oral contraceptive containing ethinyloestradiol and drospirenone. *Eur J Contracept Reprod Health Care* **5**(1), 25–34.

Inman WH, Vessey MP, Westerholm B, Engelund A. (1970) Thromboembolic disease and the steroidal content of oral contraceptives: a report to the Committee on Safety of Drugs. *Br Med J* **2**, 203–9.

International Working Group on Enhancing Patient Compliance and Oral Contraceptive Efficacy (1993) Consensus statement. *Br J Fam Plann* **18**, 126–9.

Jick H, Jick S, Gurewich V, Myers MW, Vasilakis C. (1995) Risk of idiopathic cardiovascular death and non-fatal venous thromboembolism in women using oral contraceptives with differing progestogen components. *Lancet* **346**, 1589–93.

Jick H, Kaye JA, Vasilakis-Scaramozza C, Jick SS. (2000) Risk of venous thromboembolism among users of third generation oral contraceptives compared with users of oral contraceptives with levonorgestrel before and after 1995: cohort and case-control analysis. *Br Med J* **321**, 1190–5.

Korver T, Dieben T, Vree M, Van Muijen AE, Vromans L, Van Der Sanden A, Van Osta G. (1998) A double-blind study comparing the contraceptive efficacy, acceptability and safety of two progestogen-only pills containing desogestrel 75 micrograms/day or levonorgestrel 30 micrograms/day. Collaborative Study Group on the Desogestrel-containing Progestogen-only Pill. *Eur J Contracept Reprod Health Care* **3**(4), 169–78.

Korver T, Klipping C, Heger-Mahn D, Duijkers I, van Osta G, Dieben T. (2005) Maintenance of ovulation inhibition with the 75-microg desogestrel-only contraceptive pill (Cerazette) after scheduled 12-h delays in tablet intake. *Contraception* **71**(1), 8–13.

Laffan M, Tuddenham E. (1998) Assessing thrombotic risk. *Br Med J* **317**, 520–3.

Lande RE. (1995) *New era for injectables.* Population Reports, Series K, No. 5. Baltimore: Johns Hopkins School of Public Health.

Laurel A, Stadtmauer A, Wong BC, Oehninger S. (2002) Should patients with polycystic ovary syndrome be treated with metformin? *Hum Reprod* **17**(12), 3016–25.

Lewis MA, Spitzer WO, Heinemann LAJ, MacRae KD, Bruppacher R. (1997) Lowered risk of dying of heart attack with third generation pill may offset risk of dying of thromboembolism. *Br Med J* **515**, 679–80.

Lidegaard O, Edstrom B, Kreiner S. (1998) Oral contraceptives and venous thromboembolism: a case control study. *Contraception* **57**, 291–301.

Luukkainen T. (1991) The levonorgestrel-releasing intrauterine device. *Ann NY Acad Sci* **626**, 43–9.

Machin SJ, Mackie IJ, Guillebaud J. (1995) Factor V Leiden mutation, venous thromboembolism and combined oral contraceptive usage. *Br J Fam Plann* **21**, 13–14.

Martinelli I, Sacchi E, Landi G, Taioli E, Duca F, Mannucci PM. (1998) High risk of cerebral-vein thrombosis in carriers of the prothrombin-gene mutation and in users of oral contraceptives. *N Engl J Med* **338**, 1793–7.

Medicines Control Agency. (1999) Combined oral contraceptives containing desogestrel or gestodene and the risk of venous thromboembolism. *Curr Problems Pharmacovigilance* **25**.

Mills A, Edwards IR. (1999) Venous thromboembolism and the pill. The combined oral contraceptive pill – are poor communication systems responsible for loss of confidence in this contraceptive method? *Hum Reprod* **14**(1), 7–10.

Mills A, Wilkinson C, Fotherby K. (1998) Can a change in screening and prescribing practice reduce the risk of venous thromboembolism in women taking the combined oral contraceptive pill? *Br J Fam Plann* **23**, 112–15.

Poulter NR, Chang CL, Farley TMM, Marmot MG, Meirik O. (1999) Effect on stroke of different progestagens in low oestrogen dose oral contraceptives. *Lancet* **354**, 301–2.

Provan D, O'Shaughnessy DF. (1999) Recent advances in haematology. *Br Med J* **318**, 991–4.

Redmond GP, Olson WH, Lippman JS, Kafrissen ME, Jones TM, Jorizzo JL. (1997) Norgestimate and ethinyl estradiol in the treatment of acne vulgaris: a randomized, placebo-controlled trial. *Obstet Gynecol* **89**(4), 615–22.

Rice C, Killick SR, Dieben T, Coehlingh Bennink H. (1999) A comparison of the inhibition of ovulation achieved by desogestrel 75 mcg and levonorgestrel 30 mcg daily. *Hum Reprod* **14**(4), 982–5.
Rosendaal FR. (1999) Venous thrombosis: a multicausal disease. *Lancet* **353**, 1167–73.
Royal College of General Practitioners (1967) Oral contraception and thromboembolic disease. *J R Coll Gen Pract* **13**, 267–79.
Seaman HE, de Vries CS, Farmer RDT. (2003) Differences in the use of combined oral contraceptives amongst women with and without acne. *Hum Reprod* **18**(3), 515–21.
Spitzer WO. (1997) The 1995 pill scare revisited: anatomy of a non-epidemic. *Hum Reprod* **12**(11), 2347–57.
Spitzer WO. (1998) Thromboembolism and the pill: the saga must end. *Hum Reprod* **13**(5), 1117–18.
Spitzer WO, Lewis MA, Heinemann LAJ, Thorogood M, MacRae KD on behalf of the Transnational Research Group on Oral Contraceptives and the Health of Young Women (1996) Third generation oral contraceptives and risk of venous thromboembolic disorders: an international case-control study. *Br Med J* **312**, 83–8.
Stadel BV. (1981) Oral contraceptives and cardiovascular disease. *N Engl J Med* **305**, 612–18.
Suissa S, Blais L, Spitzer W, Cusson J, Lewis M, Heinemann L. (1997) First time use of newer oral contraceptives and risk of venous thromboembolism. *Contraception* **56**, 141–6.
Szarewski A. (2000) Historical review of the combined oral contraceptive pill and injectable progestogens. *Br J Fam Plann* **26**(1), 10–11.
Szarewski A, Mansour D. (1999) The 'pill scare': responses of authorities, doctors, and patients using oral contraception. *Hum Reprod Update* **5**(6), 627–32.
Tanis BC, van den Bosch MAAJ, Kemmeren JM *et al.* (2001) Oral contraceptives and the risk of myocardial infarction. *N Engl J Med* **345**(25), 1787–93.
United Kingdom Committee on Safety of Medicines (1995) Risk of venous thromboembolism and the combined oral contraceptive pill. Statement from the Clinical and Scientific Committee of the Faculty of Family Planning and Reproductive Health Care, 15 December 1995.
Van Vloten WA, van Haselen CW, van Zuuren EJ, Gerlinger C, Heithecker R. (2002) The effect of 2 combined oral contraceptives containing either drospirenone or cyproterone acetate on acne and seborrhoea. *Cutis* **69**(4S), 2–15.
Vandenbroucke JP, van der Meer JM, Helmerhorst FM, Rosendaal FR. (1996) Factor V Leiden: should we screen oral contraceptive users and pregnant women? *Br Med J* **313**, 1127–30.
Vessey MP. (1989) The Jeffcott Lecture, 1989. An overview of the benefits and risks of combined oral contraceptives. In: Mann RD (ed.), *Oral contraceptives*

and breast cancer: the implications of the present findings for informed consent and informed choice. New York/London: Parthenon, pp. 121–35.
Vessey MP. (2001) Oral contraceptive failures and body weight: findings in a large cohort study. *J Fam Plann Reprod Health Care* **27**(2), 90–1.
Vessey MP, Doll R. (1968) Investigation of relation between use of oral contraceptives and thromboembolic disease. *Br Med J* **2**, 199–205.
Vessey MP, Mant D, Smith A, Yeates D. (1986) Oral contraceptives and venous thromboembolism: findings in a large prospective study. *Br Med J* **292**, 526.
WHO Collaborative Study of Cardiovascular Disease and Steroid Hormone Contraception. (1995) Effects of different progestogens in low oestrogen oral contraceptives on venous thromboembolism. *Lancet* **346**, 1582–8.
WHO Task Force on Postovulatory Methods of Fertility Regulation. (1998) Randomised controlled trial of levonorgestrel versus the Yuzpe regimen of combined oral contraceptives for emergency contraception. *Lancet* **352**, 428–33.

INDEX

Note: page numbers in *italics* refer to figures and boxed material